G.Y. Naroo

HEART MILES - Bevond Pheidippides

G.Y. Naroo

HEART MILES - Beyond Pheidippides

LAP LAMBERT Academic Publishing

Publisher:
LAP LAMBERT Academic Publishing
is a trademark of
Dodo Books Indian Ocean Ltd. and OmniScriptum S.R.L publishing group

120 High Road, East Finchley, London, N2 9ED, United Kingdom
Str. Armeneasca 28/1, office 1, Chisinau MD-2012, Republic of Moldova, Europe
Managing Directors: Ieva Konstantinova, Victoria Ursu
info@omniscriptum.com

Printed at: see last page
ISBN: 978-3-659-80926-2

HEART MILES------------------------------------
Beyond Pheidippides

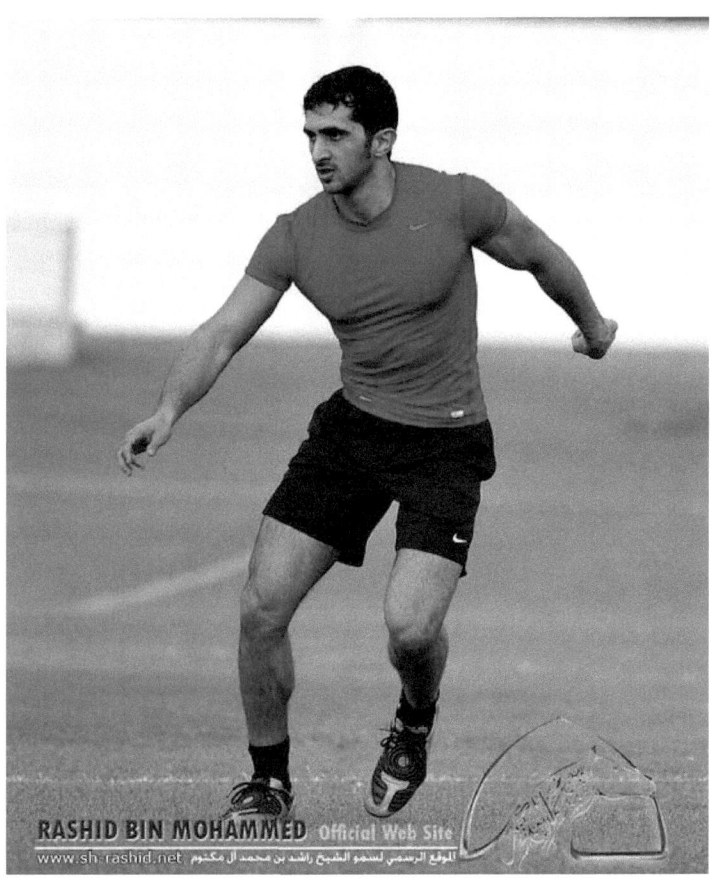

HEART MILES----------------------------------
Beyond Pheidippides

AUTHOR

Dr G Y Naroo
BSc (Hons), MBBS, MRCP (UK), FRCP (Glasg), FRCP (Ire),
MRCS A&E (Edin)
Consultant Physician - ED Trauma Centre, Rashid Hospital Dubai
Senior Lecturer - Dubai Medical College, Dubai
Senior instructor - American College of Surgeons, American Heart Association &
NAEMT

CONTRIBUTORS

1. Dr Zafar Khan
2. Dr Wajahat Zafar Khan
3. Dr Bina Naseem
4. Dr Tanveer Yadgir
5. Dr Omer Al Skaf
6. Dr Zulfiqar Ali
7. Dr Ahmad Sajjad
8. Dr Anis Ahmad
9. Dr Anas

FOREWORD

Essence of cardiac markers in marathon striders is a unique book giving in depth account on the diagnostic dilemma of cardiac markers in marathon runners. The book is a must read for internists, physicians, sport physicians and cardiologists alike.

Dr G Y Naroo is a consultant in emergency medicine at the Rashid Hospital, Dubai, UAE. A fitness freak himself, he has been in forefront of mobilizing the healthcare workers to participate in annual Dubai Marathon. His position as emergency consultant gives him an enviable opportunity to take initial care of patients in a busy emergency department. He has combined these experiences of marathon and emergency care to create this book.

The department of cardiology at Rashid Hospital is a nodal center for management of acute coronary syndrome patients in Dubai and its acute coronary syndrome program is accredited by Joint Commission International, USA. The department has been in forefront of education on the optimal use of cardiac markers in early identification and management of ACS patients.

We are confident that this book will become an essential part of learning about cardiac markers in marathon runners.

Dr Fahad Baslaib   Dr S K Agarwal
Consultant Cardiologist   Consultant Cardiologist
& HOD

DEDICATION

Dedicated to His Highness Sheikh Mohammad Bin Rashid Al Maktoom Prime minister, vice President and ruler of Dubai for his tireless passion for the sports that is a continuous inspiration to every one living in this country. As a sport person His Highness has always been involved in encouraging the people for these healthy activities irrespective of age, sex and nationality. We owe him a lot of gratitude.

Also dedicated to HH Sheikh Rashid bin Mohammed bin Rashid Al Maktoom for achieving honors in International endurance events, his role in the advancement of sports, and his perseverance for better health and happiness, Inspiring Dubai to be a Heart Safe City. You will always be missed and remembered.

HEART MILES----------------------------------
                                Beyond Pheidippides

ACKNOWLEDGEMENTS

We would like to express our gratitude to all those who provided support directly or otherwise, talked things over, read, wrote, offered comments, allowed us to follow their input and assisted in editing, proof reading and design.

We would like to thank Rashid Hospital Emergency Pathology Department for its support in collecting blood samples.

Our special thanks to Dr Ali Redha In charge medical Team for his kind supervision & encouragement.

Thanks to Dr Moin Fikree Clinical Director who has always been a source of inspiration.

Special thanks to Dr Fahad Head of Cardiology and Dr Agarwal Consultant Cardiologist Rashid Hospital for their expert opinions on the subject from conception to completion of the book.

Thanks to Mr --------------- our publisher who encouraged us.

Last but not the least, we beg forgiveness of all those who have been with us over the course of the year whose names we have failed to mention.

GY Naroo

HEART MILES-------------------------------------
                                       Beyond Pheidippides

TABLE OF CONTENTS:

HEART MILES------------------------------------
Beyond Pheidippides

INTRODUCTION:

The marathon is a long-distance running event with an official distance of 42.195 kilometers (26 miles and 385 yards) [1], that is usually run as a road race. The origin dates back to the time of a Greek messenger Pheidippides who was sent from the battlefield of Marathon to Athens to announce that the Persians has been defeated in the Battle of Marathon [2], which took place in August or September, 490 BC [3]. This endurance sports being greatly applauded has undergone a lot of research work due to the fact that it poses many health risks which can happen during and after running a marathon.

Running a distance of 26.2 miles surely inflicts the human body with an immense physiological stress which requires cardiorespiratory, endocrine and neuromuscular systems to function at their maximum optimum level, which in the long run can compromise the performance of these systems. A study published in 1996[4] found that the risk of fatal heart attack during or up to 24 hours after a marathon was approximately 1 in 50,000 over an athlete's racing career[5].

There have been many physiological and pathological implications on cardiac status of an athlete for which many studies have been done so far. The findings of such studies can help runners to evaluate their health status before and after running a marathon so that precautionary measures can be taken to avoid any harmful and fatal incidents.

Cardiac markers being the indicators of cardiac damage can be greatly influenced by running a marathon. Many studies have shown the risks of marathon running on cardiac health of an athlete. In 2006, a study was carried out on 60 non-elite marathon runners which revealed that, in that sample of 60 people, runners who had done less than 56km (35mi) per week of training before the race were most likely to show some heart damage or dysfunction, while runners who had done more than 72km (45mi) per week of training beforehand showed fewer or no heart problems [6]. In 2010, a study showed that running a marathon can reduce the function of more than half the segments in the heart's main pumping chamber, but other parts of heart will take over. Full recovery is within three months or less. The fitter the runner the less the effect [7]. The estimated risk of sudden death from jogging is one death per 396,000 man-hours of jogging and

6

Beyond Pheidippides

one death per 215,000 man-hours of running a marathon [8, 9]. The additional risk of cardiac arrest with exercise may be greater than 56- to 100- fold during or after strenuous exertion, even though the exercise reduces the overall life-time risk and is therefore beneficial[10, 11].

Cardiac markers can be helpful in evaluation of an athlete as part of the pre-participation screening or as part of the work up in case of any red flag in history, physical examination or other relevant investigations.

Marathon RUN is an attitude run, finishing 43 KM when I look insight of the thousands of runners beyond top professional runners and question comes?

Is a runner competing with other runners!!!!----	**NO**
Is a runner competing for time!!!!--------------	**NO**
Is a runner competing for the distance----------	**TRUE**

Having said that is human anatomy/ physiology /circulation & psychology could optimize this overstretch RUN!!!
As clinician perspective, we have tried to answer these questions bring possible research together of cardiac markers in marathon runners.

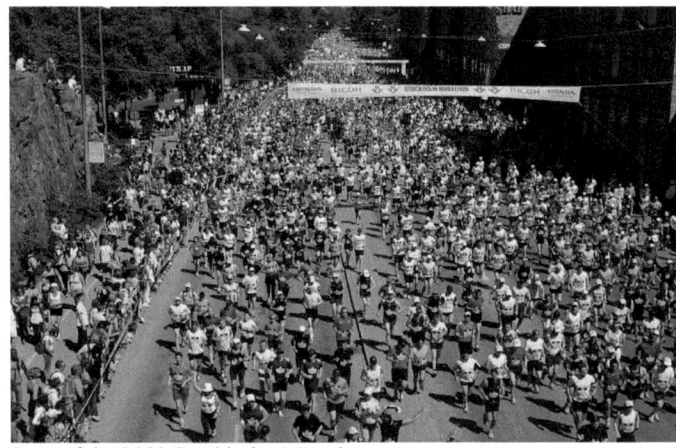

Start of the 2009 Stockholm Marathon.

Beyond Pheidippides

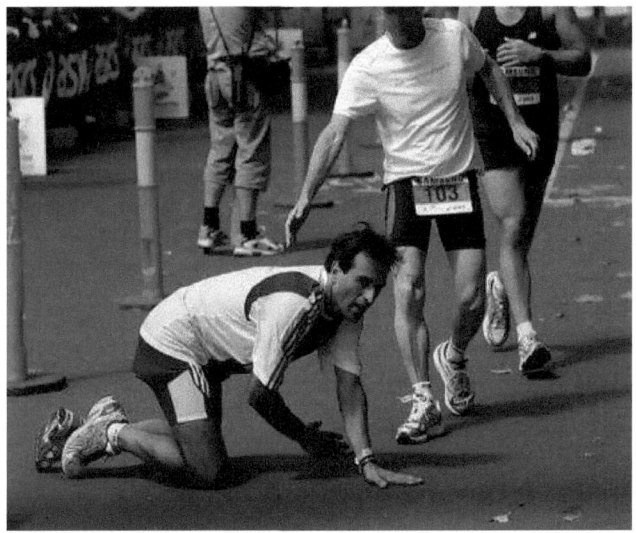

A competitor collapses just prior to the finish line of the 2006 Melbourne Marathon.

HEART MILES-----------------------------------
Beyond Pheidippides

Brief History:

As we know the marathon running originated when Greek messenger known as Pheidippides was sent to announce the victory of Athens over Persians. Pheidippides ran the 40km from Marathon to Athens, where he proclaimed the famous words "rejoice, we conquer", after which he promptly dropped dead, making him the first anecdotal case of sudden cardiac death in a marathoner [12].

Then later on, the first official Olympic marathon was run in 1896. In the commemoration of Pheidippides, Greeks relived the history of their victory by running the same distance of 40km from Marathon to Athens.

In 1908, London Olympics, the distance of the marathon was lengthened to 26.2 miles (42.195km), which took off at Windsor Castle and would finish in front of the Royal Arena so that Her Highness could watch the finish. In 1921, this distance was recognized as official marathon distance.

Death of the first runner has been brought into question by modern scholars [13], however, history has been repeating itself in the same manner as many cases of sudden deaths have been reported in few marathon runners every year. Due to this fact, many theories and studies have been documented in literature. The boldest theory regarding marathon running was made by Dr. Tom Bassler, who suggested that the stress of running a marathon built immunity to the development of fatty deposits within coronary arteries [14]. At the same conference, Bassler's claim was refuted with four documented cases of marathon runners who died from coronary artery disease [15]. History has another evidence of famous marathoner Jim Fixx, who having a strong positive family history had strong faith in Bassler's theory, ultimately died of a heart attack in the middle of the run in 1984. His faith in Bassler's theory may be why Fixx ignored chest pains while he ran, hoping they would eventually go away if he kept on running [16]. Later on autopsy revealed 100 percent and 80 percent blockage in two coronary arteries respectively and signs of previous infarctions.

A few studies have looked for signs of heart damage immediately following and for hours after completing a marathon [17, 18, 19]. Cardiac markers were raised to sub

Beyond Pheidippides

threshold levels indicating minute damage to the heart as compared to the high values of markers elevated in heart attack. However, Green found extensive damage to the heart, but no coronary artery disease, in a 44 year old marathon runner who collapsed after 24 miles of a marathon and later died [20].

Why risk profiling for cardiac status of a runner is important---

Neilan found mildly impaired heart function that persisted for one month [21].This study was carried out in post marathon runners. In order to carry out researches on marathon runners, we need to know and understand that professional marathoners have a completely different cardiac anatomy and physiology which mimics pathological patterns in otherwise non-athletes. In order to prevent fatal cardiac incidents among athletes, we need to change our approach and start risk profiling through many means for instance; through study of athlete's physiology and anatomy, emphasis on specific history, physical examination, relevant investigations. This book will be dealing with the *specifics of Cardiac markers in Marathon Runners* along with other germane areas pertinent to the subject.

References:

1. IAAF Competition Rules for Road Races. International Association of Athletics Federations. International Association of Athletics Federations. 2009. Retrieved 1 November 2010.
2. Retreats — Athens. Jeffgalloway.com. Retrieved 22 August 2009.
3. The Moon and the Marathon, Sky & Telescope. Skytonight.com (19 July 2004). Retrieved on 18 April 2013.
4. Risk for sudden cardiac death associated with marathon running. Retrieved 13 December 2008.
5. American Family Physician: Sudden death in young athletes: screening for the needle in a haystack". Aafp.org. Retrieved 22 August 2009.
6. Banking Miles: marathons dangerous for your heart?". Bankingmiles.blogspot.com. Retrieved 22 August 2009.
7. Doheny, Kathleen. (28 October 2010) Running a marathon can impact heart for months. Usatoday.com. Retrieved on 18 April 2013.

8. Thompson PD, Funk EJ, Carleton RA, Sturner WQ. Incidence of death during jogging in Rhode Island from 1975 through 1980. JAMA 1982;247:2535-8.

9. Maron BJ, Poliac LC, Roberts WO. Risk for sudden cardiac death associated with marathon running. J Am Coll Cardiol 1996;28:428-31.

10. Cobb LA, Weaver WD. Exercise: a risk for sudden death in patients with coronary artery disease. J Am Coll Cardiol 1986;7:215-9.

11. Siscovick DS, Weiss NS, Fletcher RH, et al. The incidence of primary cardiac arrest during vigorous exercise. N Engl J Med 1984;311:874-7.

12. Lovett C. Olympic marathon: a centennial history of the Games' most storied race. Westport, CT: Greenwood Publishing Group; 1997.

13. Martin, D.E., and R.W.H. Gynn. 2000. The Olympic Marathon: The History and Drama of Sport's Most Challenging Event. Champaign, Illinois; Human Kinetics.

14. Bassler, T.J. 1977. Marathon running and immunity to atherosclerosis. Annals of the New York Academy of Sciences 301:579-592.

15. Noakes, T., L. Opie, W. Beck, J. McKechnie, A. Benchimol, and K. Desser. 1977. Coronary heart disease in marathon runners. Annals of the New York Academy of Sciences 301:593-619.

16. Plymire, D.C. 2002. Running, heart disease, and the ironic death of Jim Fixx. Research Quarterly for Exercise and Sport 73(1):38-46.

17. Kratz, A., K.B. Lewandrowski, A.J. Siegel, K. Y. Chun, J.G. Flood, E.M. Van Cott, and E. Lee-Lewandrowski. 2002. Effect of marathon running on hematologic and biochemical laboratory parameters, including cardiac markers. American Journal of Clinical Pathology 118:856-863.

18. Siegel, A.J., M. Sholar, J. Yang, E. Dhanak, and K.B. Lewandrowski. 1997. Elevated serum cardiac markers in asymptomatic marathon runners after competition: Is the myocardium stunned? Cardiology 88:487-491.

19. Lucia, A.,L. Serratosa, A. Saborido, J. Pardo, A. Boraita, M. Moran, F. Banders, A. Megias, and J.L. Chicharro. 1999. Short-term effects of marathon running: No evidence of cardiac dysfunction. Medicine and Science in Sports and Exercise 31(10):1414-1421.

20. Green, L.H., S.I. Cohen, and G. Kurland. 1976. Fatal myocardial infarction in marathon racing. Annals of Internal Medicine 84(6):704-706.

Beyond Pheidippides

21. Neilan, T., D. Yoerger, P. Douglas, J. Marshall, E. Halpern, D. Lawlor, M. Picard, and M.Wood. 2006. Persistent and reversible cardiac dysfunction among amateur marathon runners. European Heart Journal 27(9):1079-1084.

Beyond Pheidippides

SECTION 1. PATHOPHYSIOLOGICAL ASPECTS

1.1.   RISE IN TROPONIN IN MARATHON RUNNERS:

The role of exercise in the prevention, management, and treatment of cardiovascular disease has been well described [1]. Although regular exercise training reduces cardiovascular disease risk, recent studies have documented elevations in biomarkers consistent with cardiac damage (i.e., cardiac troponin [cTn]) after bouts of prolonged exercise in apparently healthy individuals [2, 3, 4 and 5]. cTns are highly specific markers of myocardial cell damage[6] and are central to the diagnosis of acute coronary syndrome(ACS) [7]. cTn elevation is also apparent in conditions that result in significant cardiac stress in the absence of obstructive coronary disease [8]. Even minor elevations in cTn confer worse prognosis in patients across a wide spectrum of disease processes [9, 10 and 11]. Accordingly, increased cTn levels after exercise can generate clinical concern and subject athletes to unnecessary hospital admissions and invasive procedures [12].

Beyond Pheidippides

Structure and function:

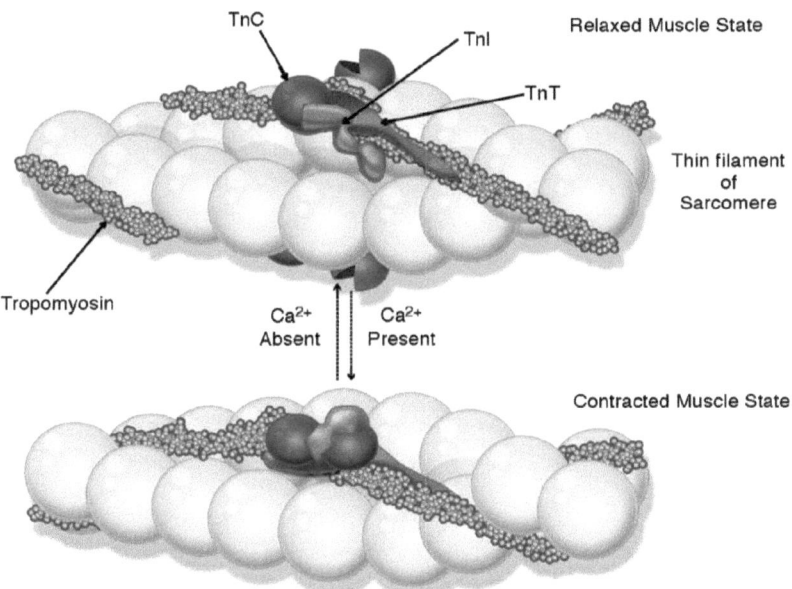

Figure illustrating location of cardiac troponin I (TnI), cardiac troponin T (TnT), and troponin C (TnC) in relation to actin and tropomyosin.

The myocardial sarcomeric unit consists of 7 actin monomers, double stranded tropomyosin and a troponin complex [6]. The troponin complex consists of three subunits namely as:

1-Troponin T (TnT)
2-Troponin C (TnC)
3-Troponin I (TnI)

Troponin T is responsible for anchoring the troponin complex to tropomyosin strand, Troponin C is responsible for binding calcium ions which are released from sarcoplasmic reticulum, and Troponin I which has a strong affinity for actin inhibits hydrolysis of adenosine triphosphate which when cleaves provide the power for

14

contraction of the muscle. The globular head of troponin complex comprises of Troponin C, Troponin I and C-Terminal portion of Troponin T, whereas the tail of troponin complex has N-Terminal portion of Troponin T. Most (>90%) cTn is bound to tropomyosin on the thin filament of myofibril, with the remainder accounted for by a small unbound cytosolic pool [13].

Ontogeny and cardiospecificity:

Cardiac and skeletal muscle share a common developmental pathway but originate from different embryonic precursors [14]. TnT and TnI both are found in cardiac as well as skeletal muscle. cTnT and cTnI representing for cardiac(c) isoforms and sTnT and sTnI representing for skeletal(s) isoforms, each expressed by separate genes.3 distinct isoforms of troponin T representing for cardiac, fast skeletal and slow skeletal are expressed simultaneously. A fourth isoform, fetal cTnT, is transiently expressed [15] but is ultimately absent in adults [16]. Studies have reported that the cTnT gene is expressed in low concentrations in cardiac and skeletal muscle until mid-fetal development, at which point the cTnT gene is upregulated in cardiac myocytes and suppressed in skeletal myocytes [17]. Conversely, cTnI is not expressed in the myocardium during fetal development and is only detectable in adult cardiac tissue [18]. In the absence of cTnI, slow twitch sTnI dominates during fetal cardiac development until ultimately replaced by cTnI during the first 9 months of life [19].

Release kinetics and Routine clinical use:

After an ischemic insult to myocardium, cTn is released in circulation in a biphasic manner. Initial release of troponin is followed by a larger sustained release. This larger release reaches its peak in serum concentration at 12-24h.The initial rise in serum cTn seems to originate from the cytosolic pool with the later rise attributable to release of bound cTn [20]. Although debated, the initial release of cytosolic cTn with ischemia might be due to changes in myocardial membrane permeability, whereas the release of bound cTn requires proteolytic degradation and cellular necrosis [21].The half -life of cTnT in the circulation is 120min [22].

15

HEART MILES---------------------------------
Beyond Pheidippides

The sensitivity and specificity of cardiac troponins is far superior to old biomarkers including lactate dehydrogenase, creatine kinase, creatine kinase-myocardial band and myoglobin in detecting myocardial injury. The cTn measurement is a component of the universal definition of acute myocardial infarction [7].

The release of cTn due to pathologic myocardial damage can be divided into 3 mechanistic categories [23];
1- Because of ruptured coronary arterial plaque and coronary occlusion.
2-Because of the increased myocardial oxygen demand with less myocardial oxygen supply.
3- Because of non-ischemic cardiac injury in which cTn release is caused by direct damage to the myocardium, including blunt trauma [24], penetrating trauma [25], myocarditis [26], or drug and toxin-induced cardio-toxicity [27].

The release of cardiac troponins in a healthy individual after exercise cannot be elaborated by the above mentioned pathophysiology.

Biomarkers of Myocardial Injury in Exercise:

History:

Early reports of post-exercise elevations in serum concentrations of the myocardial band isoform of creatine kinase (CK-MB) [28] raise the concerns that such activities can be responsible for cardiac injury. However, elevations in serum CK-MB after prolonged exercise lack specificity for the detection of cardiomyocyte damage [29]. The CK-MB is increased in the skeletal muscle of distance runners [30] perhaps because of increases in satellite cells, which repair injured skeletal muscle [31]. Thus, in the investigation of exercise-induced cardiac injury, attention shifted from CK-MB to cTn, a highly specific marker of cardiac muscle damage, even in the presence of significant skeletal muscle breakdown [32].

Beyond Pheidippides

cTn elevation after exercise:

After the development of second and third generation cTnT assays, with recombinant human cTnT as the reference, we are able to detect cTn release precisely in response to cardiomyocyte damage. Competitive athletic events demanding increased cardiac output, heart rate, and systolic blood pressure for several hours in conjunction with elevations in reactive oxygen species, altered pH and increased core temperature can hypothetically damage cardiomyocytes. Troponin levels from participants in marathon-distance [4, 33, 34 and 35] and ultra-distance foot races [36 and 37], triathlons [3 and 38], and dedicated cycling events [39 and 40] have each been studied.

Several studies have reported no significant post-exercise cTn elevations [29, 41 and 42], but the majority of data document statistically significant cTn increases after exercise [34, 35, 36, 43 and 44]. Variations in serum concentrations of cTn after prolonged endurance exercise can possibly be due to the differences in the fitness levels of participants, the type or duration of exercise, the timing of the post exercise sample, the troponin assay used, and the detection limit used to define a positive cTn. A recent meta-analysis examined data from 26 studies and found that post-exercise cTn concentrations exceeded the assay's lower limit in approximately half of participants [44]. Many studies have provided important information, including the observation that cTn is increased after prolonged walking in a non-athletic population and that the magnitude of increase is related to exercise intensity and cardiovascular pathology [45]. Recently, 9 highly trained male triathletes were studied during participation in a simulated half-ironman event (1.9km pool swim, 90-km cycle ergometry, 21.1-km treadmill run), and cTnT increases were observed in 4 of the athletes [46]. More recently, cTnT concentrations have been compared in 13 adolescent male runners (age 14.8 +/- 1.6 years) after 4 constant load treadmill runs of varying duration (45 or 90 min) and intensity (80% or 100% ventilatory threshold) [47]. The highest cTnT median concentration was found among the participants who had the longest exercise duration and highest exercise intensity.

cTn elevation and myocardial function:

Many investigators have carried out non -invasive testing of myocardial function along with cTn testing. Neilan et al. [4] measured cTnT and performed echocardiography 20 min after the race in non-elite participants completing a Boston Marathon. Results showed that increases in cTnT were associated with reductions in right ventricular contractility. Whereas, George et al. [37] found no correlation between post-race troponin elevations and echocardiographic parameters of left ventricular function.

On the other hand, Mousavi et al. [35] reported elevated cTnT in 14 marathon finishers with concomitant echocardiographic evidence of transient right ventricular systolic and biventricular diastolic dysfunction. After one week, MRI showed no evidence of persistent damage. But a case report of myocardial fibrosis in a veteran endurance athlete [48] warrants the need for more research.

Potential Mechanisms of cTn release after exercise:

Increased membrane permeability:

Increased membrane permeability might be responsible for the release of cytosolic cTn. Such an increase in membrane permeability might be due to increased mechanical stress on the cardiomyocytes [49], increased production of oxidative radicals [50], or altered acid base balance [51]. These physiologic processes have been documented in skeletal muscle exposed to exercise and seem to play an important role in adaptive skeletal muscle hypertrophy [49 and 52]. Mechanical stimuli might produce transient disruptions of the myocardial plasma membrane, termed "cell wounds" [53], making it possible that exercise-induced cTn release reflects the activation of cellular cascades that result in cardiac hypertrophy [54].

An alternative mechanism for exercise-induced cTn release is the stimulation of integrins by myocardial stretch [55]. Integrins act as bidirectional signaling molecules and are involved in cardiac re-modeling with pressure overload or after myocardial infarction [56]. Stimulating stretch-responsive integrins mediates the transport of intact

Beyond Pheidippides

cTn molecules out of viable cardiomyocytes [57]. The release of cTnI from necrotic cardiac myocytes is different from the release of cTn because of stimulated integrins.

Recently, Feng et al. [58] have shown in a rat model the degradation of cTnI with increasing preload, in the absence of ischemia, suggesting that myocardial stretch per se can degrade cTn. Thus it can be possible that the release of cTn degraded products instead of intact troponin can be the result of myocardial stretching without any evidence of ischemia.

References:

1. I.M. Lee, J.E. Manson, C.H. Hennekens, R.S. Paffenbarger Jr Body weight and mortality: A 27-year follow-up of middle-aged men JAMA, 270 (1993), pp. 2823–2828

2. N. Middleton, K. George, G. Whyte, D. Gaze, P. Collinson, R. Shave Cardiac troponin T release is stimulated by endurance exercise in healthy humans J Am Coll Cardiol, 52(2008), pp. 1813-1814

3. N. Rifai, P.S. Douglas, M. O'Toole, E. Rimm, G.S. Ginsburg Cardiac troponin T and I, echocardiographic [correction of electrocardiographic] wall motion analyses, and ejection fractions in athletes participating in the Hawaii Ironman Triathlon Am J Cardiol, 83 (1999), pp. 1085–1089

4. T.G. Neilan, J.L. Januzzi, E. Lee-Lewandrowski, et al. Myocardial injury and ventricular dysfunction related to training levels among nonelite participants in the Boston marathon Circulation, 114 (2006), pp. 2325–2333

5. R.E. Shave, G.P. Whyte, K. George, D.C. Gaze, P.O. Collinson Prolonged exercise should be considered alongside typical symptoms of acute myocardial infarction when evaluating increases in cardiac troponin T Heart, 91 (2005), pp. 1219–1220

6. P.O. Collinson, F.G. Boa, D.C. Gaze Measurement of cardiac troponins Ann Clin Biochem, 38 (2001), pp. 423–449

7. K. Thygesen, J.S. Alpert, H.D. White Universal definition of myocardial infarction J Am Coll Cardiol, 50 (2007), pp. 2173–2195

Beyond Pheidippides

8. A. Jeremias, C.M. Gibson Narrative review: alternative causes for elevated cardiac troponin levels when acute coronary syndromes are excluded Ann Intern Med, 142 (2005), pp. 786–791

9. K. Thygesen, J.S. Alpert, H.D. White, et al. Universal definition of myocardial infarction Circulation, 116 (2007), pp. 2634–2653

10. S. James, P. Armstrong, R. Califf, et al. Troponin T levels and risk of 30-day outcomes in patients with the acute coronary syndrome: prospective verification in the GUSTO-IV trial Am J Med, 115 (2003), pp. 178–184

11. C. Becattini, M.C. Vedovati, G. Agnelli Prognostic value of troponins in acute pulmonary embolism: a meta-analysis Circulation, 116 (2007), pp. 427–433

12. G. Whyte, N. Stephens, R. Senior, et al. Treat the patient not the blood test: the implications of an increase in cardiac troponin after prolonged endurance exercise Br J Sports Med, 41 (2007), pp. 613–615 discussion 615

13. J. Bleier, K.P. Vorderwinkler, J. Falkensammer, et al. Different intracellular compartmentations of cardiac troponins and myosin heavy chains: a causal connection to their different early release after myocardial damage Clin Chem, 44 (1998), pp. 1912–1918

14. J.H. Mar, R.C. Iannello, C.P. Ordahl Cardiac troponin T gene expression in muscle Symp Soc Exp Biol, 46 (1992), pp. 237–249

15. C.J. Sutherland, K.A. Esser, V.L. Elsom, M.L. Gordon, E.C. Hardeman Identification of a program of contractile protein gene expression initiated upon skeletal muscle differentiation Dev Dyn, 196 (1993), pp. 25–36

16. P.A. Anderson, N.N. Malouf, A.E. Oakeley, E.D. Pagani, P.D. Allen Troponin T isoform expression in humans: A comparison among normal and failing adult heart, fetal heart, and adult and fetal skeletal muscle Circ Res, 69 (1991), pp. 1226–1233

17. T.A. Cooper, C.P. Ordahl A single troponin T gene regulated by different programs in cardiac and skeletal muscle development Science, 226 (1984), pp. 979–982

18. J.E. Humphreys, P. Cummins Regulatory proteins of the myocardium: Atrial and ventricular tropomyosin and troponin-I in the developing and adult bovine and human heart J Mol Cell Cardiol, 16 (1984), pp. 643–657

19. S. Sasse, N.J. Brand, P. Kyprianou, et al. Troponin I gene expression during human cardiac development and in end-stage heart failure Circ Res, 72 (1993), pp. 932–938

20. A.H. Wu, Y.J. Feng, R. Moore, et al. Characterization of cardiac troponin subunit release into serum after acute myocardial infarction and comparison of assays for troponin T and I: American Association for Clinical Chemistry Subcommittee on cTnI Standardization Clin Chem, 44 (1998), pp. 1198–1208

21. A.H. Wu, L. Ford Release of cardiac troponin in acute coronary syndromes: ischemia or necrosis? Clin Chim Acta, 284 (1999), pp. 161–174

22. H.A. Katus, A. Remppis, T. Scheffold, K.W. Diederich, W. Kuebler Intracellular compartmentation of cardiac troponin T and its release kinetics in patients with reperfused and nonreperfused myocardial infarction Am J Cardiol, 67 (1991), pp. 1360–1367

23. P.O. Collinson, P.J. Stubbs Are troponins confusing? Heart, 89 (2003), pp. 1285–1287

24. G.J. Fulda, F. Giberson, D. Hailstone, A. Law, M. Stillabower An evaluation of serum troponin T and signal-averaged electrocardiography in predicting electrocardiographic abnormalities after blunt chest trauma J Trauma, 43 (1997), pp. 304–310 discussion 310-2

25. M. Keel, C. Meier Chest injuries—what is new? Curr Opin Crit Care, 13 (2007), pp. 674–679

26. M.A. Baig, S. Ali, M.U. Khan, et al. Cardiac troponin I release in non-ischemic reversible myocardial injury from parvovirus B19 myocarditis Int J Cardiol, 113 (2006), pp. E109–E110

27. D.C. Gaze, P.O. Collinson Cardiac troponins as biomarkers of drug- and toxin-induced cardiac toxicity and cardioprotection Expert Opin Drug Metab Toxicol, 1 (2005), pp. 715–725

28. A.J. Siegel, L.M. Silverman, B.L. Holman Elevated creatine kinase MB isoenzyme levels in marathon runners: Normal myocardial scintigrams suggest noncardiac source JAMA, 246 (1981), pp. 2049–2051

29. F.S. Apple, M.A. Rogers, W.M. Sherman, D.L. Costill, F.C. Hagerman, J.L. Ivy Profile of creatine kinase isoenzymes in skeletal muscles of marathon runners Clin Chem, 30 (1984), pp. 413–416

30. P.D. Thompson, F.S. Apple, A. Wu Marathoner's heart? Circulation, 114 (2006), pp. 2306–2308

31. A.J. Siegel, L.M. Silverman, W.J. Evans Elevated skeletal muscle creatine kinase MB isoenzyme levels in marathon runners JAMA, 250 (1983), pp. 2835–2837

32. R. Shave, E. Dawson, G. Whyte, et al. The cardiospecificity of the third-generation cTnT assay after exercise-induced muscle damage Med Sci Sports Exerc, 34 (2002), pp. 651–654

33. A. Mingels, L. Jacobs, E. Michielsen, J. Swaanenburg, W. Wodzig, M. van Dieijen-Visser Reference population and marathon runner sera assessed by highly sensitive cardiac troponin T and commercial cardiac troponin T and I assays Clin Chem, 55 (2009), pp. 101–108

34. E.B. Fortescue, A.Y. Shin, D.S. Greenes, et al. Cardiac troponin increases among runners in the Boston Marathon Ann Emerg Med, 49 (2007), pp. 137–143 143.e1

35. N. Mousavi, A. Czarnecki, K. Kumar, et al. Relation of biomarkers and cardiac magnetic resonance imaging after marathon running Am J Cardiol, 103 (2009), pp. 1467–1472

Beyond Pheidippides

36. R.E. Shave, E. Dawson, G. Whyte, et al. Evidence of exercise-induced cardiac dysfunction and elevated cTnT in separate cohorts competing in an ultra-endurance mountain marathon race Int J Sports Med, 23 (2002), pp. 489–494

37. K. George, R. Shave, D. Oxborough, et al. Left ventricular wall segment motion after ultra-endurance exercise in humans assessed by myocardial speckle tracking Eur J Echocardiogr, 10 (2009), pp. 238–243

38. L. Tulloh, D. Robinson, A. Patel, et al. Raised troponin T and echocardiographic abnormalities after prolonged strenuous exercise—the Australian Ironman Triathlon Br J Sports Med, 40 (2006), pp. 605–609

39. J. Scharhag, M. Herrmann, A. Urhausen, M. Haschke, W. Herrmann, W. Kindermann Independent elevations of N-terminal pro-brain natriuretic peptide and cardiac troponins in endurance athletes after prolonged strenuous exercise Am Heart J, 150 (2005), pp. 1128–1134

40. G. Neumayr, R. Pfister, G. Mitterbauer, G. Eibl, H. Hoertnagl Effect of competitive marathon cycling on plasma N-terminal pro-brain natriuretic peptide and cardiac troponin T in healthy recreational cyclists Am J Cardiol, 96 (2005), pp. 732–735

41. A.J. Siegel, J.J. Stec, I. Lipinska, et al. Effect of marathon running on inflammatory and hemostatic markers Am J Cardiol, 88 (2001), pp. 918–920

42. G. Lippi, F. Schena, G.L. Salvagno, et al. Influence of a half-marathon run on NT-proBNP and troponin T Clin Lab, 54 (2008), pp. 251–254

43. A.J. Saenz, E. Lee-Lewandrowski, M.J. Wood, et al. Measurement of a plasma stroke biomarker panel and cardiac troponin T in marathon runners before and after the 2005 Boston marathon Am J Clin Pathol, 126 (2006), pp. 185–189

44. R. Shave, K.P. George, G. Atkinson, et al. Exercise-induced cardiac troponin T release: a meta-analysis Med Sci Sports Exerc, 39 (2007), pp. 2099–2106

45. T. Eijsvogels, K. George, R. Shave, et al. Effect of prolonged walking on cardiac troponin levels Am J Cardiol, 105 (2010), pp. 267–272

46. R. Shave, E. Dawson, G. Whyte, K. George, D. Gaze, P. Collinson Altered cardiac function and minimal cardiac damage during prolonged exercise Med Sci Sports Exerc, 36 (2004), pp. 1098–1103

47. F. Fu, J. Nie, T.K. Tong Serum cardiac troponin T in adolescent runners: effects of exercise intensity and duration Int J Sports Med, 30 (2009), pp. 168–172

48. W.J. Rowe Extraordinary unremitting endurance exercise and permanent injury to normal heart Lancet, 340 (1992), pp. 712–714

49. P.L. McNeil, R. Khakee Disruptions of muscle fiber plasma membranes: Role in exercise-induced damage Am J Pathol, 140 (1992), pp. 1097–1109

50. A. Goette, A. Bukowska, D. Dobrev, et al. Acute atrial tachyarrhythmia induces angiotensin II type 1 receptor-mediated oxidative stress and microvascular flow abnormalities in the ventricles Eur Heart J, 30 (2009), pp. 1411–1420

51. E. Hultman, K. Sahlin Acid-base balance during exercise Exerc Sport Sci Rev, 8 (1980), pp. 41–128

52. W.J. Evans, J.G. Cannon The metabolic effects of exercise-induced muscle damage Exerc Sport Sci Rev, 19 (1991), pp. 99–125

53. M.S. Clarke, R.W. Caldwell, H. Chiao, K. Miyake, P.L. McNeil Contraction-induced cell wounding and release of fibroblast growth factor in heart Circ Res, 76 (1995), pp. 927–934

54. J. Scharhag, A. Urhausen, G. Schneider, et al. Reproducibility and clinical significance of exercise-induced increases in cardiac troponins and N-terminal pro brain natriuretic peptide in endurance athletes Eur J Cardiovasc Prev Rehabil, 13 (2006), pp. 388–397

55. A. Koller, W. Schobersberger Post-exercise release of cardiac troponins J Am Coll Cardiol, 53 (2009), p. 1341 author reply 1341–2

56. R.S. Ross, T.K. Borg Integrins and the myocardium Circ Res, 88 (2001), pp. 1112–1119

57. M.H. Hessel, D.E. Atsma, E.J. van der Valk, W.H. Bax, M.J. Schalij, A. van der Laarse Release of cardiac troponin I from viable cardiomyocytes is mediated by integrin stimulation Pflugers Arch, 455 (2008), pp. 979–986

58. J. Feng, B.J. Schaus, J.A. Fallavollita, T.C. Lee, J.M. Canty Jr Preload induces troponin I degradation independently of myocardial ischemia Circulation, 103 (2001), pp. 2035–2037

HEART MILES------------------------------------

Beyond Pheidippides

1.2. RISE IN CPK AND CKMB IN MARATHON RUNNERS:

CPK and CKMB:

CPK and CKMB have been affected by many factors causing variations in their serum values, especially acute and chronic physical activity. Due to these variations, the use of the measurements of these biomarkers when evaluating heart or skeletal muscle injury should not be relied upon completely, especially in case of an athlete.

Introduction:

CPK being a large IM protein is found in two or more than two forms in human body, which are made up of two subunits namely as M and B.

Following are the three naturally occurring forms of CPK present in humans:
1) CK-MM (skeletal muscle)
2) CK-MB (cardiac muscle)
3) CK-BB (brain)
CK-MM:
-99% of CPK activity in skeletal muscle
-70% to 85% of CPK activity in cardiac muscle
CK-MB:
-1% of CPK activity in skeletal muscle
-15% to 30% of CPK activity in cardiac muscle
CK-BB:
The third iso-enzyme, CK-BB, is active primarily in brain with some activity in such other organs as the lungs, spleen, pancreas and kidneys [1, 2].

CPK is mainly responsible for forming adenosine tri-phosphate (ATP=energy) which is used mainly in heart and skeletal muscle myofibrils during muscle contraction. Thus, during a short term or long term exercise, CPK is needed for maintenance of energy in the muscle cell during contraction.

Beyond Pheidippides

Due to the restrictive size of the molecules of these large proteins (CPK, CK-MM, CK-MB), these are only released into bloodstream in muscle membrane injury. Therefore, these proteins are being extensively used as diagnostic biomarkers in case of myocardial and skeletal muscle injury and disease. However, physical activity having major influence on serum CPK and CK-MB activity, the serum cut offs for diagnosing cardiac muscle injury(myocardial infarction) and disease should be approached with caution.

Acute Exercise:

Unaccustomed or novel physical exercise involving varying types of muscle contractions has been shown to produce skeletal muscle damage [3].Concentric (muscle tension and muscle shortening) and isometric (muscle tension and no muscle shortening) muscle contractions have been shown to initiate increases in serum CPK activity, but to a much lesser extent than eccentric (muscle lengthening and contractile process shortening) contractions [4, 5].

Friden et al [6] found that subjects who exercised eccentrically had increases in serum CPK activity but that those who exercised concentrically or isometrically had no increases in serum CPK. Schwane et al [7] found a 351% increase in serum CPK activity after an eccentric exercise session of downhill running (for 45 minutes. at 57% of maximal oxygen consumption, and on a 10% grade) and no change in serum CPK after an exercise session of running on a level surface.

Newham et al [8] conducted a bench-stepping test in which one leg always stepped eccentrically and the other concentrically. Pain and tenderness developed within 8 hours in the eccentric leg and peaked at 48 hours. Maximum strength decreased in the eccentric leg, which recovered 24 hours after exercise. In the concentrically exercised leg soreness did not develop, and the leg recovered its strength over a shorter period. Newham et al [9] used the same bench-stepping protocol and found that eccentric exercise resulted in pain, disruption of the sarcomere architecture, alterations in cell membrane permeability resulting in an efflux of IM enzymes (CPK, CK-MB), and degeneration of muscle fibers with infiltration of macrophages. Other examples of eccentric exercise that results in muscle injury and thus an increase in serum CPK and CK-MB include eccentric hamstring and forearm curls [10, 11].

Tiidus and Ianuzzo [12] demonstrated that although duration affects serum CPK activity, the intensity of exercise is of greater importance in causing serum CPK elevations and delayed muscle soreness. They found that when total work was kept constant, the high-intensity, short-duration group exhibited significantly greater serum CPK activity than the low-intensity, long-duration group.

Three of the hypothesized mechanisms of muscle injury are [13]:
1) Imbalance of calcium influx resulting in reduced mitochondrial function.
2) An increase in intracellular pH, which causes a destabilization of the lysosomal membranes.
3) Macrophage infiltration that enhances protease activity.

Long term (training) exercise:

Siegel et al [14] found post-race elevations in serum CPK and CK-MB for 15 Boston Marathon runners. There was a 21 fold increase in serum CPK activity 24 hours post-race which returned to normal as of pre-race levels after 4 weeks. Apple et al [15] compared serum CPK and CK-MB activities in subjects after a marathon and after an acute myocardial infarction. Both the markers were found to be elevated at 1,24,48,72 hours post-race. Peak CK-MB activity was found to be higher in marathoners as compared to those of myocardial infarction patients. However, relative percentages were 7% and 7.2% respectively.

Apple et al [16] found an increase in skeletal muscle CK-MB with exercise training. The proposed mechanism was that muscle fibre necrosis due to training sessions cause regeneration of new muscle fibres from these necrosed muscle fibres which results in increased CK-MB. This increased CK-MB causes an increase in the serum proportion of CK-MB with muscle injury. These results have also been found in eccentric exercises like bench stepping, forearm flexion, and downhill running after repeated sessions. However, the effects of these types of exercises are lessened on subsequent sessions of similar exercise [17].A single session of downhill running will reduce post exercise serum CPK activity and post exercise muscle soreness after similar runs for up to 9 weeks after the last downhill run [18]. Subsequent training sessions result in continued

Beyond Pheidippides

decrease in serum enzyme activities. This suggests some type of adaptive process in either the rate of enzyme leakage or in the rate of enzyme clearance from the blood [19].

Newham et al [17] suggested three explanations for this observed training effect:
1) A change in the pattern of muscle fiber recruitment, which on subsequent bouts of exercise would spare damaged fibers.
2) Muscle fiber adaptation making them more resistant to the stress of exercise.
3) Certain types of contractions (eccentric) that damage particular fibers at the end of the cycle of growth and replacement.

Gender and physical activity:

Women exhibit lower serum CPK activity at rest compared with men [20]. Shumate et al [20] observed differences in untrained men and women performing bicycle egometry exercise at 50% maximal oxygen consumption. Results showed a five-fold increase in serum CPK activity from 122mU/mL to 664mU/mL as compared to women showing only two-fold increase from 72mU/mL to 152mU/mL.

It has been hypothesized that variations in muscle fiber recruitment or variations in muscle mass account for the differences seen between men and women [21, 22]. Another mechanism has been mentioned in literature. The role of estrogen and its derivatives has been implicated in the reduction in CPK efflux in women as compared to men [23].

Age and physical activity:

After 30 years of age, physiologic functions decline from 0.75% to 1% per year [24]. Gale and Murphy [25], using a cross-sectional sample of adults, computed that the increases in serum CPK activity were approximately 3 U/L per decade. Smith et al [26] examined resting serum CPK activity in 625 healthy women and found a marked increase in resting CPK activity with increasing age. Meltzer [27] also reported increased serum CPK activity with advancing age.

Beyond Pheidippides

Schneider et al [28] found that excessive exercise placed an overabundance of stress on an already declining muscular system, as evidenced by increased CPK and CK-MB activity after exercise.

After all these results, they concluded that the use of absolute or relative CPK activity for diagnostic purposes with respect to aging patients must be used with caution.

Variability of serum CPK and CK-MB activity:

There is an extreme variability in serum activities of these enzymes. For example, Newham et al [8] found that subjects who performed an eccentric exercise session had CPK activities ranging from 500 U/L to 34,500 U/L.

The temperature of the stored samples is another factor which affects the serum activities of these enzymes. For example, in a serum stored at 37 degree Celsius, approximately 30%-40% of the original CPK activity disappears within 8 hours [29]. The final CPK activity value is also affected according to the different levels of sensitivity of the assay technique being used. For example, the CPK and CK-MB analysis techniques of Sigma Diagnostics (St Louis, Missouri) have a coefficient of variation of 6.2% to 10%, which must be taken into account when using serum CPK and CK-MB activities for diagnosing myocardial and skeletal muscle injury [29].

Conclusion:

According to the mentioned evidences about the effects of physical activity, gender and age on serum CPK and CK-MB, a greater caution is needed when relying on the use of serum CPK and CK-MB as diagnostic and evaluative biomarkers for muscle injury.

References:

1) DM Dawson, IH Fine Creatine kinase in human tissues Arch Neurol, 16 (1967), pp. 175–180

2) H Lang Creatine Kinase Isoenzymes: Pathophysiology and Clinical Application Springer-Verlag New York, Inc, New York (1981)

3) RB Armstrong Muscle damage and endurance events Sports Med, 3 (1986), pp. 370–381

4) R Buckley-Bleiler, RJ Maughan, PM Clarkson, et al. Serum creatine kinase activity after isometric exercise in premenopausal and postmenopausal women Exp Aging Res, 15 (1989), pp. 195–198

5) J Friden, M Sjostrom, B Ekblom Myofibrillar damage following intense eccentric exercise in man Int J Sports Med, 4 (1983), pp. 170–176

6) J Friden, PN Sfakianos, AR Hargens Blood indices of muscle injury associated with eccentric muscle contractions J Orthop Res, 7 (1989), pp. 142–145

7) JA Schwane, SR Johnson, CB Vandenakker, et al. Delayed-onset muscular soreness and plasma CPK and LDH activities after downhill running Med Sci Sports Exerc, 15 (1983), pp. 51–56

8) DJ Newham, DA Jones, RH Edwards Large and delayed plasma creatine kinase changes after stepping exercise Muscle Nerve, 6 (1983), pp. 380–385

9) DJ Newham, DA Jones, EJ Tolfree, et al. Skeletal muscle damage: A study of isotope uptake, enzyme efflux and pain after stepping J Appl Physiol Occup Physiol, 55 (1986), pp. 106–112

10) CM Schneider, KD Pai, ME Zoller Creatine kinase, aspartate aminotransferase, and perceived soreness following exercise-induced muscle injury Med Exerc Nutr Health, 1 (1992), pp. 281–286

11) MP Miles, CM Schneider Creatine kinase MB may be elevated in healthy young women after submaximal eccentric exercise J Lab Clin Med, 122 (1993), pp. 197–201

12) PM Tiidus, CD Ianuzzo Effects of intensity and duration of muscular exercise on delayed soreness and serum enzyme activities Med Sci Sports Exerc, 15 (1983), pp. 461–465

13) RB Armstrong Initial events in exercise-induced muscular injury Med Sci Sports Exerc, 22 (1990), pp. 429–435

14) AJ Siegel, LM Silverman, RE Lopez Creatine kinase elevations in marathon runners: Relationship to training and competition Yale J Biol Med, 53 (1980), pp. 275–279

15) FS Apple, MA Rogers, WM Sherman, et al. Comparison of serum creatine kinase and creatine kinase MB activities post marathon race versus post myocardial infarction Clin Chem Acta, 138 (1984), pp. 111–118

16) FS Apple, MA Rogers, WM Sherman, et al. Profile of creatine kinase isoenzymes in skeletal muscle of marathon runners Clin Chem Acta, 30 (1984), pp. 413–416

17) DJ Newham, DA Jones, PM Clarkson Repeated high force eccentric exercise: Effects on muscle pain and damage J Appl Physiol, 63 (1987), pp. 1381–1386
18) WC Byrnes, PM Clarkson, JS White, et al. Delayed onset muscle soreness following repeated bouts of downhill running J Appl Physiol, 59 (1985), pp. 710–715

19) TD Noakes Effect of exercise on serum enzyme activities in humans Sports Med, 4 (1987), pp. 245–267

20) JB Shumate, MH Brooke, JE Carroll, et al. Increased serum creatine kinase after exercise: A sex-linked phenomenon Neurology, 29 (1979), pp. 902–904

21) MA Rogers, GA Stull, FS Apple Creatine kinase isoenzyme activities in men and women following a marathon race Med Sci Sports Exerc, 17 (1985), pp. 679–682

22) LP Novak, GW Tillery Relationship between serum creatine phosphokinase and body composition Hum Biol, 49 (1977), pp. 375–380

23) GJ Amelink, PR Bar Exercise-induced muscle protein leakage in the rat: Effects of hormonal manipulation J Neurol Sci, 76 (1986), pp. 61–68

24) GA Brooks, TD Fahey Exercise Physiology: Human Bioenergetics and Its Applications Macmillan Publishing Co, New York (1985)

25) AN Gale, EA Murphy The use of serum creatine phosphokinase in genetic counseling for Duchenne muscular dystrophy J Chron Dis, 32 (1979), pp. 639–651

26) I Smith, RA Elton, WHS Thomson Carrier detection in X linked recessive (Duchenne) muscular dystrophy: Serum creatine phosphokinase values in premenarchal, menstruating, postmenopausal and pregnant normal women Clin Chem Acta, 98 (1979), pp. 207–216

27) HY Meltzer Factors affecting serum creatine phosphokinase levels in the general population: The role of race, activity, and age Clin Chem Acta, 33 (1971), pp. 165–172

28) CM Schneider, MA Rogers, JW Lampe, et al. Serum creatine kinase isoenzyme measurements in master male and female marathon runners Sports Med Training Rehab, 3 (1992), pp. 237–242

29) Sigma Chemical Company Biochemicals Organic Compounds for Research and Diagnostic Reagents Sigma Chemical Co, St Louis (1993)

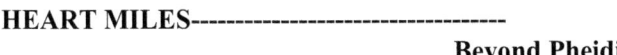

Beyond Pheidippides

1.3. ATHLETE'S HEART:

The athlete heart is a term that has been used for many years by physicians and laymen to describe the cardiovascular effects of long term conditioning observed in highly trained competitive athletes (1-4). Physiologic responses to prolonged training include increased stroke volume and decreased heart rate under resting conditions; with long term training there is enhanced extraction of oxygen by peripheral skeletal muscle and reduced blood lactate levels associated with increased maximal arterio-venous oxygen difference and increased maximal oxygen consumption (5-11). The clinical manifestations of the "athlete heart syndrome" , as originally described, include sinus bradycardia at rest, a soft systolic murmur, audible third and fourth heart sounds, cardiomegaly on chest X-ray and a variety of alterations in the scalar electrocardiogram (1).

Initially, heart enlargement in athletes was identified largely by physical examination and chest radiography, or inferred from electrocardiographic patterns suggestive of left ventricular enlargement or hypertrophy (1-19). For the past 4 decades a number of echocardiographic studies (2, 3, 10, 20-59) have been performed in a variety of athletic populations. Since the advent of M-mode echocardiography, cardiac dimensions and functions have been defined more accurately.

As we know that echocardiographic studies provide a comparison of cardiac dimensions between trained athletes and sedentary subject. Though the values for dimensions in trained athletes are usually only slightly increased compared with those in control subjects and rarely exceed the normal range (60, 61).

Cardiac structure and dimensions:

Left Ventricular Mass:

Echocardiographic studies have shown that left ventricular mass with an average increase of 46% was present in athletes than in control subjects. Such echocardiographic estimates of mass are usually derived employing the formula of Troy et al. (62), which incorporates end-diastolic left ventricular transverse dimension, and posterior free wall

Beyond Pheidippides

thickness, or that of Devereaux and Reichek (63). The increased left ventricular mass identified in most athletes is not related solely to body size; that is, the "athlete heart" is not larger than normal because the athlete may have a larger than normal body size; cardiac dimensions still differ significantly between athletes and control subjects when normalized for body surface area or weight (9, 20, 27,36, 39,40,46-48). Maximal oxygen consumption, probably the single most objective indicator of a training effect, is also increased in athletes (average 38%) (23,27,28,30, 31,35,36,38,43,47,48).

Left Ventricular Cavity:

(Figure 1)
Figure 1.M-mode echocardiograms recorded at the level of the mitral valve (MV) showing cardiac dimensions in two trained athletes. A, From a 19 year old male football player showing findings typical of an endurance athlete. The ventricular septum (VS) and posterior left ventricular free wall (PW) are both mildly thickened (12 mm each) and the left ventricular cavity is slightly increased in transverse dimension (LVIDct) (56 mm); the right ventricular (RV) cavity is of normal size. LV = left ventricle; MV = mitral valve. B, From an 18 year old lacrosse player showing more substantial enlargement of ventricular cavities; the left ventricular transverse end-diastolic dimension (LVIDct) is 60 mm and the right ventricular (RV) dimension is 32 mm. In contrast to the athlete shown in A, ventricular septal (VS) and posterior (PW)

Beyond Pheidippides

thicknesses are normal (1O mm each). Calibration dots are IO mm apart in both panels.

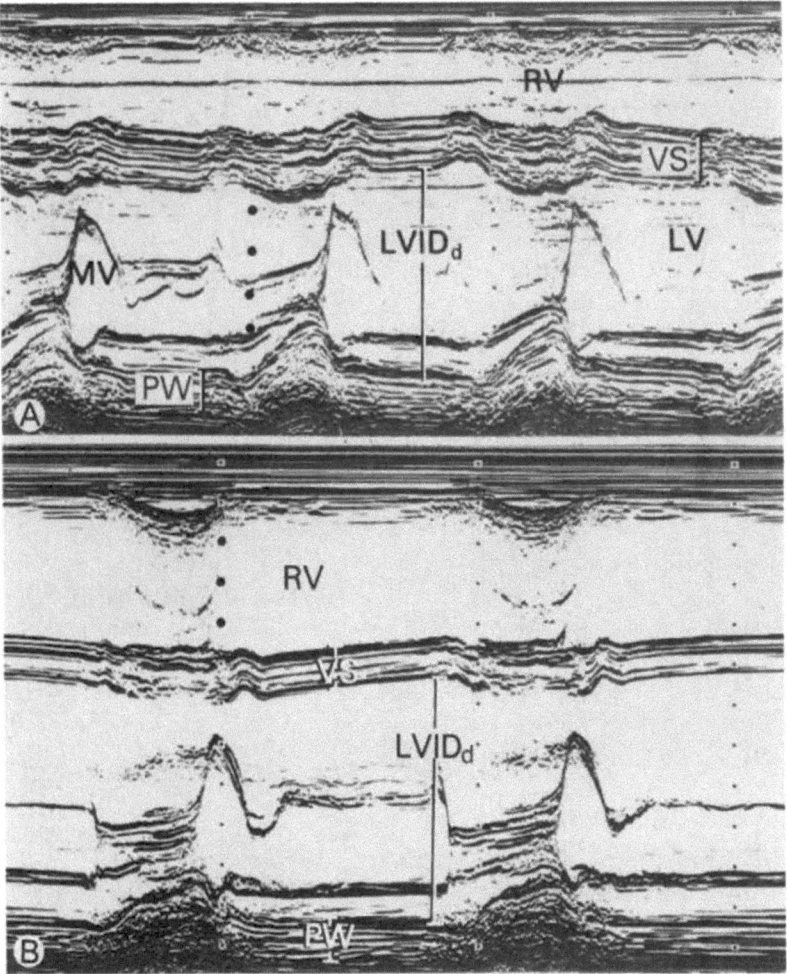

As shown in figure 1, due to an increase in transverse end diastolic dimension of left ventricle, athletes have increased left ventricular mass but this mass usually does not cross the normal upper limit in adults without any cardiac disease. This increased dimension is relatively mild as compared to those of diseased hearts producing left ventricular cavity dilation. Echocardiographic data has shown an increase of 10% in this dimension which is equivalent to 33% difference in left ventricular volume as compared to matched sedentary control subjects. Average left ventricular transverse end diastolic dimension in athletes is almost 54mm and maximal is 64mm, however normal athlete's heart usually does not exceed the dimension of more than 60mm. Left ventricular end-systolic dimension is usually increased in athletes compared with control subjects(22,25-27,29,31,36,38,43,47), although this difference is usually mild and has achieved statistical significance in only some investigations(27,29,31,36,43,47).

Left Ventricular Wall Thickness:

Ventricular septal and posterior left ventricular free wall thickness is increased with average values of 10.4 and 10.6mm respectively. However, wall thickness has rarely exceeded 14mm with the maximal reported thickness as 16mm.these average values of thicknesses are within the accepted normal values but are 14%(septal) and 19%(free wall) more than the values reported for matched sedentary control subjects.

M mode echo has shown a symmetric septal and free wall thickness (normal septal/free wall ratio of <1.3), however, some reports (21, 25, 50) have described a small number of athletes with an increased septal/free wall ratio suggesting an asymmetric pattern of left ventricular hypertrophy. Only Shapiro (50) reported a significant proportion (28%) of athletes with a septal/free wall ratio greater than 1.3.But he used two dimensional echo for measurements, which is less desirable for quantitative measurement of wall thickness.

Right Ventricular Cavity:

Studies have shown an average increase of 22mm in right ventricular dimension (maximum 33) as compared to the control subjects (17mm), a difference of 24%. This increase can be attributed to increase in ventricular mass induced by long term conditioning.

Beyond Pheidippides

Left Atrial Size:

Studies have shown the enlargement of left atrium in athletes. However the cause unknown, it has been proposed that the enlargement in size is a reflection of impaired ventricular function.

Determinants of increased cardiac dimensions in athletes:
All available echocardiographic data has shown that the increase in left ventricular wall thickness and cavity in particular is truly a direct response of training in athletes. However, it is also possible that such cardiac alterations are not produced solely by intense training, but are due, in part, to a genetic predisposition that exists before training (10). Although this issue has not been resolved, it would seem unlikely that increased left ventricular mass is importantly determined by genetic factors in most athletes because of the facility and rapidity with which change in the activity level can alter the magnitude of left ventricular mass (28, 38, 43). It is also necessary to consider the possibility that the increase in left ventricular transverse dimension commonly present in athletes is partially due to training-induced bradycardia and the concomitant prolongation of the diastolic filling period (10). However, Hirshleifer et al. (64) found that in normal subjects very small changes in left ventricular dimension accompanied marked changes in heart rate (induced by atropine). Therefore, bradycardia cannot be the only reason for increased left ventricular cavity size in athletes.

Relation of cardiac structural changes to the nature of athletic conditioning:

The findings of several investigations (20,33,34,39,40,45,46,49,52),particularly those of Morganroth et al. (20) and Longhurst et al. (39,40), suggest that the precise alterations in cardiac structure in athletes may differ depending on the type of training activity undertaken.

For instance, athletes of isotonic endurance sports have more volume load thus resulting in increased ventricular cavity dimension without any significant change in wall thickness. In contrast, athletes who do weight training sports (isometric or static) have more pressure load thus resulting in increased left ventricular wall thickness without any significant change in cavity dimension.

Beyond Pheidippides

In addition, Longhurst et al (39, 40) demonstrated that although both isotonic and isometric training increased left ventricular mass, they did so in different ways relative to lean body mass. The increase in left ventricular mass in case of isotonic training was disproportionately greater than the increase in skeletal muscle mass, whereas, isometric training resulted only in increased left ventricular mass in proportion to the increase in skeletal muscle mass.

The different effects of isotonic and isometric exercise on cardiac dimensions are not always clear-cut; some investigators have not found significant differences in cardiac morphology between athletes participating in each of these two types of activity (41).

Changes in left ventricular dimensions and mass associated with conditioning and deconditioning:

Conditioning:

Many studies have shown that the initiation of strenuous physical exercise program can result in the development of moderate degree of left ventricular hypertrophy very quickly (within weeks or months).

Ehsani et al (28) used M-mode echocardiography to study eight competitive swimmers at the conclusion of a period of deconditioning (2 to 7 months) and then serially for a subsequent 9 week period of intense training. Left ventricular end diastolic dimension increased by about 10% (as compared to deconditioned state) after one week of training and then remained constant for 8 weeks. Posterior wall thickness gradually increased, significant increases of about 7%(as compared to deconditioned state) were not there for 5 weeks and as a result posterior wall thickness remained constant.

Similarly, Wieling et al. (38), in studies on collegiate oarsmen, found relatively rapid increases in left ventricular mass shortly after initiation of training. After 4 months of training, there was a significant increase in left ventricular end diastolic dimension and ventricular septal thickness, whereas, posterior wall thickness increased after 7 months of training.

Deconditioning:

Ehsani et al. (28) showed that within 1 week of total cessation of training, a significant decrease in left ventricular diastolic dimension (8%), posterior wall thickness (15%) and calculated left ventricular mass (27%) occurred ; these changes became even more marked over the next 2 weeks (overall change of 9,25 and 38% respectively).

Fagard et al. (43) studied 12 competitive bicyclists and also found a decrease in left ventricular mass associated with detraining, manifested by a reduction in ventricular septal and posterior left ventricular wall thicknesses, but without significant change in left ventricular end diastolic dimension.

Shapiro and Smith (59) reported regression in left ventricular mass after a 6 week period of detraining in 10 non-athletes who had previously participated in a standardized 6 week exercise program.

Shapiro (50) also observed normal cardiac dimensions in a group of deconditioned ex-athletes 5 or more years after they had ceased competitive activities.

Such changes in left ventricular mass with training and detraining have been shown (23,27,28,30,31,35,36,38,43,47,48) to occur in parallel with alterations in maximal oxygen consumption. Furthermore, maximal oxygen consumption has been shown (30,36) to have a relation to the magnitude of left ventricular cavity enlargement.

Left ventricular function:

Systolic Function:

Percent fractional shortening or derived ejection fraction or velocity of circumferential fiber shortening comes in normal range among most athletes when left ventricular systolic function is assessed by M-mode echocardiography. Such measurements do not reflect the global function and considered as segmental in nature. Nevertheless, relatively mild deviations from normal left ventricular contractility have been reported (31, 43) in only two studies, both involving competitive bicyclists.

Nishimura et al. (31) found indexes of left ventricular contractility to be mildly decreased in competitive bicyclists in the 40 to 49 year old age group who had trained for most of their adult lives (an average of 27 years). Fagard et al. (43) found a significant decrease in percent fractional shortening associated with regression in left ventricular mass after 8 weeks of detraining. Because of the increase of end diastolic and end systolic dimensions in similar magnitude after long term conditioning; percent fractional shortening and ejection fraction is found to be normal in athletes. Reryth et al. (65) assessed global cardiac function in 18 competitive swimmers with radionuclide angiography before and after 6 months of training. Though left ventricular end diastolic volume was increased, ejection fraction at rest was decreased from a mean value of 73% before training to 67% after training.

Diastolic Function:

Several recent reports have described diastolic function in trained athletes using a number of non-invasive techniques, including digitized M-mode echocardiography (49), Doppler echocardiography (66) and radionuclide angiography (48). Granger et al. (48), using radionuclide angiography, found that despite a 43% increase in left ventricular mass over that of control subjects, athletes showed no alteration in left ventricular filling. Hence, unlike pathologic hypertrophy due to chronic systolic hemodynamic overload (67-71), coronary artery disease (72) or primary myocardial disease (70,71,73,74), "physiologic" left ventricular hypertrophy induced by exercise is apparently not accompanied by impaired left ventricular diastolic function. Matsuda et al. (75), using digitized M-mode echocardiography reported an augmentation of early diastolic filling with exercise in athletes.

Elite athletes:

Morganroth et al. (20) found no differences in cardiac dimensions between world class runners and shot putters and their non-elite counterparts. In addition, Underwood and Schwade (25) found no differences in cardiac morphology between elite endurance

41

runners and other competitive runners. On the other hand, Shapiro (50) reported that national standard athletes had significantly greater left ventricular wall thicknesses and mass compared with those of collegiate and recreational sportsmen. But these wall thicknesses still fall into normal range. Therefore, enhanced performance can be attributed to genetically determined body structure and function.

Childhood athletes:

The study of Allen et al. (76) in 77 competitive age-group swimmers (5 to 17 years of age) demonstrated that the morphologic changes of the athlete heart may be identified early in life, presumably because of the training regimen to which these children were exposed. There was an increased thickness of septum and both ventricular walls along with the increase in right ventricular cavity size as compared to sedentary control subjects. Left ventricular end diastolic cavity dimension was also found to be greater in 30% of athletes as compared to sedentary subjects.

Geenen et al. (77) showed that in 6 and 7 year old children (non-athletes), left ventricular posterior wall thickness and left ventricular mass increased after an 8 month aerobic exercise program. These two studies, (76,77) which show left ventricular wall thickening to usually occur in the absence of significant left ventricular cavity enlargement, differ considerably from the studies in adult endurance athletes in whom left ventricular cavity enlargement is the most consistent structural alteration (10). These differences show that training has different effects on cardiovascular system of adults and children.

Beyond Pheidippides

The athlete heart and hypertrophic cardiomyopathy:

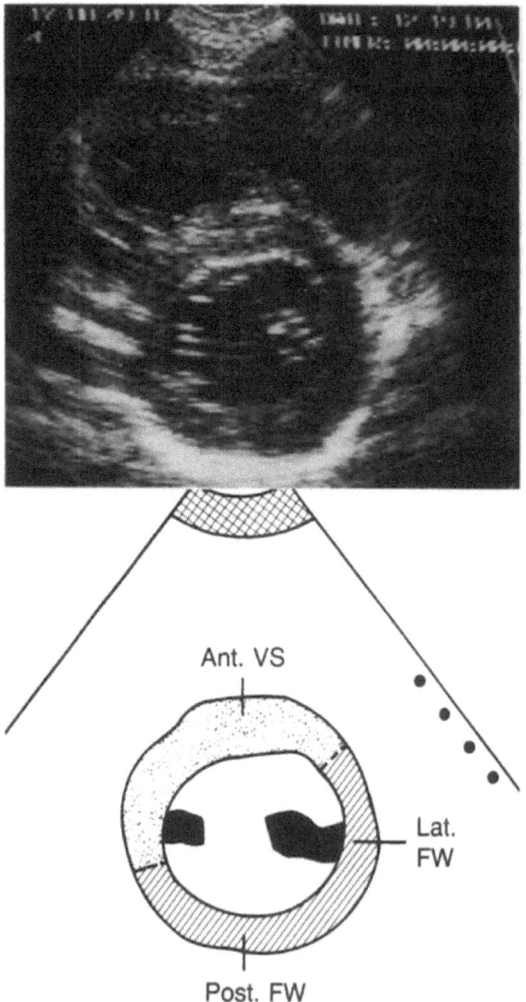

Ant. VS

Lat. FW

Post. FW

Beyond Pheidippides

Figure above. Stop-frame two-dimensional echocardiogram (at end-diastole) in the short-axis cross sectional plane from a 22 year old competitive runner. There is a relatively mild increase in thickness of the anterior ventricular septum (Ant. YS) (13 mm); other segments of the left ventricular wall appear to be of normal thickness. Left and right ventricular cavities are of normal size. Calibration dots are 10 mm apart. Lat. FW = lateral free wall; Post. FW = posterior free wall.

The athlete's heart can resemble hypertrophic cardiomyopathy. Diagnostic dilemma in evaluating athlete's heart occurs when there is a mild increase of 13-15mm in ventricular septal thickness with no dilatation of left ventricular cavity along with the absence of systolic anterior motion of the mitral valve (fig shown above). In such circumstances, it may be extremely difficult to discriminate between the 'physiologic' increase in left ventricular mass produced by athletic training and the relatively mild (but pathologic) hypertrophic cardiomyopathy (78,79); hence, such athletes appear to fall into an equivocal 'grey zone'(fig 3).

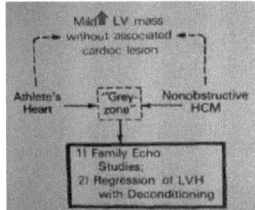

Fig 3:-Diagram summarizing the relation between the normal athlete heart, non-obstructive hypertrophic cardiomyopathy (HCM) and the heart of athletes in whom morphologic cardiac findings are intermediate between the two ("Grey-zone"). Echo = echocardiographic; LV = left ventricular; LVH = left ventricular hypertrophy; = increased.

In addition, athletes with the normal athlete heart and patients with non-obstructive hypertrophic cardiomyopathy may show a variety of similarly abnormal (or even normal) patterns on the 12 lead electrocardiogram (1-4,20-22,25,26,29,31,36-38,43,47,80-84).

This diagnostic dilemma demands an additional assembly of clinical data. For instance, because hypertrophic cardiomyopathy is often genetically transmitted (85, 86), echo studies on a relative showing morphologic dimensions of cardiomyopathy can make this diagnosis likely in an athlete. However, negative echo studies in relatives of an athlete would not definitively exclude the diagnosis of hypertrophic cardiomyopathy since this disease may occur without apparent familial transmission (85).

An additional method to differentiate between these two is prospective deconditioning of an athlete(for 3 to 6 months) to verify if left ventricular wall thickening or cavity dimension, or both, have decreased or not. The decrease in these parameters would be a result of deconditioning of athlete's heart, whereas there would not be any significant change in these parameters in case of hypertrophy due to a cardiac disease. 24 hour ambulatory monitoring can also be used for athletes falling in 'grey zone'.

Long term significance of athlete heart:

As emphasized by Oakley (87), the morphologic features of the athlete heart have been well defined with M-mode echocardiography. However, the echocardiographic observations are used to assess athlete's heart at one point in time making it difficult to assess the long term physiology of the heart, specifically the physiologic left ventricular hypertrophy of athlete's heart which may be rapidly reversible with the cessation of conditioning (28, 43).

The study of Nishimura et al. (31) suggests that persistent conditioning through middle life may progressively increase left ventricular mass after age 40 years.

Sudden Death:

Young athletes with congenital cardiovascular diseases (particularly hypertrophic cardiomyopathy) (88,89) are most commonly responsible for these catastrophes, while virtually all sudden deaths in older athletes are due to coronary heart disease (89-92).

Occasional young athletes have been reported (88,89) who died suddenly and at autopsy were found to have a moderate increase in left ventricular mass characterized by a

Beyond Pheidippides

symmetric pattern of wall thickening in the presence of non-dilated ventricular cavities, normal myocardial architecture and no evidence of genetic transmission of cardiomyopathy to relatives.

Although unlikely, but for undefined pathophysiologic reasons, athletes with idiopathic left ventricular hypertrophy represent rare malignant expressions of athlete's heart.

References

1) Gott PH, Roselle HA, Crampton RS. The athletic heart syndrome. Five-year cardiac evaluation of a champion athlete. Arch Intern Med 1968; 122:340-4

2) Raskoff WJ, Goldman S, Cohn K. The"athletic heart." Prevalence and physiological significance of left ventricular enlargement in distance runner. JAMA 1976;236:158-62

3) Crawford MH, O'Rourke RA. The athlete's heart. Adv Intern Med 1979:311-29 (Stollerman GH, ed Yearbook Medical Publication; vol 24)

4) Rost R, Hollmann W Athlete's heart-A review of its historical assessment and new aspects. Int J Sports Med 1983; 4: 147-65

5) Beckner GL, Winsor T. Cardiovascular adaptations to prolonged physical effort. Circulation 1954; 9:835-45

6) Reindell H, Roskamm H. Stem H. The heart and blood circulation in athletes. Med Welt 1960;31:1557-63

7) Bevegard S, Holmgren A, Jonsson B. Circulatory studies in well trained athletes at rest and during heavy exercise with special reference to stroke volume and the influence of body position. Acta Physiol Scand 1963;57:26-50

8) Scheuer J, Tipton CM. Cardiovascular adaptations to physical training. Annu Rev Physiol 1977;39:221-51

Beyond Pheidippides

9) Blomqvist CG, Saltin B. Cardiovascular adaptations to physical training Annu Rev Physiol 1983; 45:169-89

10) Schaible TF, Scheuer J. Cardiac adaptations to chronic exercise Prog Cardiovasc Dis 1985; 27:297-324

11) Longhurst JC, Kelly AR, Gonyea WJ, Mitchell JH. Cardiovascular responses to static exercise in distance runners and weight lifters. J Appl Physiol (Respir Environ Exerc Physiol) 1980; 49:676-83

12) Henschen S,Skilauf and Skiwettlauf. Eine medizinsche Sportstudie. Mitt Med Klinik Uppsala 1899; 2:15

13) Marach JH Physiological and pathological effects of severe exertion,marathon race, on circulatory and renal system. Arch Intern Med 1910; 5:382-405

14) Herxheimer H. Unterschungen uber die Anderung der Hergro unter dem Einflu bestinmter Sportarten. Z Klin Med 1929; 111:376-93.

15) Keys A, Friedell HL. Size and stroke of the heart in young men in relation to athletic activity. Science 1938; 88:456-8.

16) Gordon B,Levine SA,Welmaers A. A group of marathon runners with special reference to circulation. Arch Intern Med 1924; 33:425-534.

17) Klemola E. Electrocardiographic observations of 650 Finnish athletes. Ann Med Intern Fenn 1951;40 :121-32.

18) Karvonen MJ,Rautaharju P,Rousteenoja R. Heart size of champion skiers. Ann Med Intern Fenn 1957; 46:169-78.

19) Bulychev VV,Khmelevskii VA,Rutman IV. Roentgenological and instrumental examination of the heart in athletes. Klin Med (Mosk)1965; 43:108-14.

HEART MILES----------------------------------
Beyond Pheidippides

20) Morganroth J, Maron BJ, Henry WL, Epstein SE. Comparative left ventricular dimensions in trained athletes. Ann Intern Med 1975; 82:521-4.

21) Roeske WR, O'Rourke RA, Klein A, Leopold G, Karliner JS. Non-invasive evaluation of ventricular hypertrophy in professional athletes. Circulation 1976; 53:286-92.

22) Zoneraich S, Rhee JJ, Zoneraich O, Jordan D, Apple J. Assessment of cardiac function in marathon runners by graphic non-invasive techniques. Ann NY Acad Sci 1977;301:900-17.

23) Gilbert CA, Nutter DO, Felner JM, Perkins JV, Heymsfield SB, Schlant RC. Echocardiographic study of cardiac dimensions and functions in the endurance-trained athlete. Am J Cardiol 1977; 40:528-33.

24) Laurenceau JL, Turrat J, Dumesnil J. Echocardiographic findings in Olympic athletes (abstr). Circulation 1977; 56(suppl III):III-25.

25) Underwood RH, Schwade JL. Noninvasive analysis of cardiac function in elite distance runners-echocardiography, vectorcardiography, and cardiac intervals. Ann NY Acad Sci 1977; 301:297-309.

26) Parker BM, Londeree BR, Cupp GV, Dubiel JP. The noninvasive cardiac evaluation of long-distance runners. Chest 1978; 73:376-81.

27) Zeldis SM, Morganroth J, Rubler S. Response of the heart to Isotonic conditioning in female athletes. A correlation between echocardiographically determined left ventricular size and exercise performance J Appl Physiol 1978; 44:849-52.

28) Ehsani AA, Hagberg JM, Hickson RC. Rapid changes in left ventricular dimensions and mass in response to physical conditioning and deconditioning Am J Cardiol 1978; 42:52-6.

29) Ikaheimo MJ, Palatsi lJ, Takkunen JT. Noninvasive evaluation of the athletic heart: sprinters versus endurance runners. Am J Cardiol 1979; 44:24-30.

30) Blair NL, Youker JE, McDonald IG, lelinek VM. Echocardiographic assessment of cardiac chamber size and left ventricular function in aerobically trained athletes. Aust NZ J Med 1980; 10:540-7.

31) Nishimura T, Yamada Y, Kawai C. Echocardiographic evaluation of long-term effects of exercise on left ventricular hypertrophy and function in professional bicyclists. Circulation 1980; 61.832-40.

32) Heath GW, Hagberg JM, Eshani AA, Holloszy JO. A physiological comparison of young and older endurance athletes. J Appl Physiol (Respir Environ Exerc Physiol) 1981;51 :634-40.

33) Keul J, Dickhuth H-H, Simon G, Lehmann M. Effect of static and dynamic exercise on heart volume, contractility. and left ventncular dimensions. Circ Res 1981; 48(suppl l): I-162-70.

34) Dickhuth H-H, Simon G, Kindermann W, Wildberg A, Keul J. Echocardiographic studies on athletes of various sport-types and non-athletic persons. Z Kardiol 1979; 68:449-53.

35) Paulsen W, Boughner DB, Cunningham DA, Persaud JA. Left ventricular function in marathon runners: echocardiographic assessment. J Appl PhysioI (Respir Environ Exerc Physiol) 1981;51:881-6

36) Bekaert I, Pannier JL, Van De Weghe C, Van Durme JP, Clement DL, Pannier R. Non-invasive evaluation of cardiac function in professional cyclists. Br Heart J 1981;45:213-8.

37) Mumford M, Prakash R. Electrocardiographic and echocardiographic characteristics of long distance runners. Comparison of left ventricular function with age- and sex-matched controls Am J Sports Med 1981 ;9:23-8.

38) Wieling W, Borghols EAM, Hollander AP, Danner SA, Dunning AJ. Echocardiographic dimensions and maximal oxygen uptake in oarsmen during training. Br Heart J 1981; 46:190-5.

39) Longhurst JC, Kelly AR, Gonyea WJ, Mitchell JH. Chronic training with static and dynamic exercise. cardiovascular adaptation and response to exercise. Circ Res 1981; 48(suppl l):I-171-8.

40) Longhurst JC, Kelly AR, Gonyea WJ, Mitchell JH. Echocardiographic left ventricular masses in distance runners and weight lifters. J Appl Physiol (Respir Environ Exerc Physiol) 1980; 48: 154-62.

41) Snoeckx LHEH, Abeling HFM, Lambregts JAC, Schmitz JJF, Verstappen FTJ, Reneman RS. Echocardiographic dimensions in athletes in relation to their training programs. Med Sci Sports Exerc 1982; 14.428-34.

42) Rost R. The athlete's heart. Eur Heart J 1982;3(suppl A).193-8.

43) Fagard R, Aubert A, Lysens R, Staessen J, Vanhees L, Amery A. Noninvasive assessment of seasonal variations in cardiac structure and function m cyclists. Circulation 1983; 67:896-901

44) Brown S, Byrd R, Jayasinghe, Jones D. Echocardiographic characteristics of competitive and recreational weight lifters. JCU 1983; 2: 163-5

45) Sugishita Y, Koseki S, Matsuda M, Yamaguchi T, Ito l. Myocardial mechanics of athletic hearts in comparison with diseased hearts. Am Heart J 1983; 105:273-80.

46) Spirito P, Maron BJ, Bonow RO, Epstein SE. Prevalence and significance of an abnormal S-T segment response to exercise in a young athletic population. Am J Cardiol 1983;51:1663-6.

Beyond Pheidippides

47) Fagard R, Aubert A, Staessen J, VanDen Eynde E, Vanhees L, Amery A. Cardiac structure and function in cyclists and runners. Comparative echocardiographic study. Br Heart J 1984; 52: 124-9.

48) Granger CB, Karimeddini MK, Smith V-E, Shapiro HR, Katz AM, Riba AL. Rapid ventricular filling in left ventricular hypertrophy. I. Physiologic hypertrophy. J Am Coll Cardiol 1985; 5:862-8

49) Colan SD, Sanders SP, MacPherson D, Borow KM. Left ventricular diastolic function in elite athletes with physiologic cardiac hypertrophy. J Am Coll Cardiol 1985; 6:545-9.

50) Shapiro LM. Physiological left ventricular hypertrophy. Br Heart J 1984; 52:130-5.

51) Peronnet F, Ferguson RJ, Perrault H, Ricci G, Lajoie D. Echocardiography and the athlete's heart. Phys Sports Med 1981; 9:102-12.

52) Howald H, Maire R, Heirl B, Follath F. Echocardiographische Befunde bei trainierten Sportlern. Schweiz Med Wochenschr 1977; 197:1662-6.

53) DeMaria AN, Neumann A, Lee G, Fowler W, Mason DT. Alterations in ventricular mass and performance induced by exercise training in man evaluated by echocardiography. Circulation 1978; 57:237-44.

54) Wolfe LA, Cunningham DA, Rechnitzer PA, Nichol PM. Effects of endurance training on left ventricular dimensions in healthy men. J Appl Physiol (Respir Environ Exerc Physiol) 1979; 47:207-12.

55) Stein RA, Michielli D, Diamond J, Horwitz B, Krasnow N. The cardiac response to exercise training: echocardiographic analysis at rest and during exercise. Am J Cardiol 1980; 46:219-25.

56) Peronnet F, Perrault H, Cleroux J, et al. Electro- and echocardiographic study of the left ventricle in man after training. Eur J Appl Physiol 1980; 45: 125-30.

57) Kanakis C, Hickson RC. Left ventricular response to a program of lower-limb strength training. Chest 1980; 78:618-21.

58) Adams TD, Yanowitz FG, Fisher AG, Ridges JD, Lovell K, Pryor TA. Noninvasive evaluation of exercise training in college-age men.Circulation 1981;64:958-65.

59) Shapiro LM, Smith RG. Effect of training on left ventricular structure and function. An echocardiographic study. Br Heart J 1983;50:534-9

60) Gardin JM, Henry WL, Savage DD, et al. Echocardiographic measurements In normal subjects: evaluation of an adult population without clinically apparent heart disease. JCU 1979;7:439-47

61) Henry WL, Gardin JM, Ware JH. Echocardiographic measurements in normal subjects from infancy to old age. Circulation 1980; 62:1054-61

62) Troy BL, Pombo J, Rackley CE. Measurement of left ventricular wall thickness and mass by echocardiography. Circulation 1972;45:602-11

63) Devereux RB, Reichek N. Echocardiographic determination of left ventricular mass in man. Anatomic validation of the method. Circulation 1977;55:613-8

64) Hirshleifer J, Crawford M, O'Rourke RA, Karltner JS. Influence of acute alterations of heart rate and systemic arterial pressure of echocardiographic measures of left ventricular performance in normal human subjects. Circulation 1975;52:835-41.

65) Rerych SK, Scholz PM, Sabiston DC, Jones RH. Effects of exercise training on left ventricular function in normal subjects:a longitudinal study by radionuclide angiography. Am J Cardiol 1980;45:244-52

66) Finkelhor RS, Hanak LJ, Bahler RC. Diastolic function in endurance trained subjects (abstr). J Am Coll Cardiol 1985;5:540

Beyond Pheidippides

67) Eichhorn P, Grimm J, Koch R, Hess, 0, Carroll J, Krayenbuehl HP. Left ventricular relaxation in patients with left ventricular hypertrophy secondary to aortic valve disease. Circulation 1982; 65: 1395-1404

68) Inouye I, Massie B, Loge D, et al. Abnormal left ventricular filling: an early finding in mild to moderate systemic hypertension. Am J Cardiol 1984; 53: 120-6

69) Fifer MA, Borow KM, Colan SD, Lorell BH. Early diastolic left ventricular function in children and adults with aortic stenosis. J Am Coll Cardiol 1985; 5:1147-54

70) Stewart S, Mason DT, Braunwald E. Impaired rate of left ventricular filling In Idiopathic hypertrophic subaortic stenosis and valvular aortic stenosis. Circulation 1968; 37:8-14

71) Hanrath P, Mathey DG, Siegart R, Bleifeld W. Left ventricular relaxation and filling pattern in different forms of left ventricular hypertrophy. An echocardiographic study. Am J Cardiol 1980; 45: 15-23

72) Bonow RO, Bacharach SL, Green MV, et al. Impaired left ventricular diastolic filling in patients with coronary artery disease: assessment with radionuclide angiography. Circulation 1981 ; 64:315-23

73) Sanderson JE, Traill TA, St John Sutton MG, Brown DJ, Gibson DG, Goodwin JF. Left ventricular relaxation and filling in hypertrophic cardiomyopathy. an echocardiographic study. Br Heart J 1978; 40:596-601
.

74) Maron BJ, Arce J, Bonow RO, Wesley Y. Noninvasive assessment of left ventricular relaxation and filling by pulsed Doppler echocardiography in hypertrophy cardiomyopathy (abstr). Circulation 1984; 70(suppl II):II-18

75) Matsuda M, Sugishita Y, Koseki S, Ito I, Akatsuka T, Takamatsu K. Effect of exercise on left ventricular diastolic filling in athletes and nonathletes. J Appl Physiol (Respir Environ Exerc Physiol) 1983; 55: 323-8

76) Allen HD, Goldberg SJ, Sahn DJ, Schy N, Wojcik R. A quantitative echocardiographic study of champion childhood swimmers. Circulation 1977; 55: 142-5.

77) Geenen DL, Gilliam TB, Crowley D, Moorehead-Steffens C, Rosenthal A. Echocardiographic measures in 6 to 7 year old children after an 8 month exercise program. Am J Cardiol 1982; 49: 1090-5.

78) Maron BJ, Epstein SE. Hypertrophic cardiomyopathy: a discussion of nomenclature. Am J Cardiol 1979; 43:1242-4

79) Maron BJ, Gottdiener JS, Epstein SE. Patterns and significance of the distribution of left ventricular hypertrophy in hypertrophic cardiomyopathy' a Wide-angle, two-dimensional echocardiographic study of 125 patients. Am J Cardiol 1981; 48:418-28.

80) Smith WG, Cullen KJ, Thorburn I0. Electrocardiograms of marathon runners in 1962 Commonwealth Games. Br Heart J 1964; 26:469-76.

81) Van Ganse W, Versee L, Eylenbosch W, Vuylsteek K. The electrogram of athletes, comparison with untrained subjects. Br Heart J 1970; 32: 160-4

82) Hanne-Paparo N, Wendkos MH, Brunner D. T wave abnormalities in the electrocardiograms of top-ranking athletes without demonstrable organic heart disease. Am Heart J 1971 ; 81: 743-7.

83) Oakley DG, Oakley CM. Significance of abnormal electrocardiograms in highly trained athletes. Am J Cardiol 1982; 50:985-9.

84) Maron BJ, Wolfson JK, Ciro E, Spirito P. Relation of electrocardiographic abnormalities and patterns of left ventricular hypertrophy identified by two-dimensional echocardiography in patients With hypertrophic cardiomyopathy. Am J Cardiol 1983; 51:189-94

85) Maron BJ, Nichols PF, Pickle LW, Wesley YE, Mulvihill JJ. Patterns of inheritance In hypertrophic cardiomyopathy: assessment of M-mode and two-dimensional echocardiography. Am J Cardiol 1984; 53: 1087-94

86) Clark CE, Henry WL, Epstein SE. Familial prevalence and genetic transmission of Idiopathic hypertrophic subaortic stenosis. N Engl J Med 1973; 289:709-14

87) Oakley D. Cardiac hypertrophy in athletes. Br Heart J 1984; 52: 121-3

88) Maron B, Roberts WC, McAllister HA, Rosing DR, Epstein SE. Sudden death in young athletes. CIrculation 1980; 62:218-29

89) Maron BJ, Epstein SE, Roberts WC. Causes of sudden death in competitive athletes. J Am Coll Cardiol 1986; 7:204-14.

90) Thompson PD, Stern MP, Williams P, Duncan K, Haskell WL, Wood PD. Death during jogging or running. A study of 18 cases. JAMA 1979; 242:1265-7.

91) Waller BF, Roberts WC. Sudden death while running in conditioned runners aged 40 years or over. Am J Cardiol 1980; 45:1292-300.

92) Virmani R, Robinowitz M, McAllister HA. Nontraumatic death in joggers. A series of 30 patients at autopsy. Am J Med 1982; 72:874-81.

SECTION 2. LITERATURE PERSPECTIVE

2.1. CARDIAC MARKER TROPONIN T IN DUBAI MARATHON RUNNERS

Jan-Mar. 2014, Volume 11, No 1 (Serial No. 93) pp. 14-18. Journal of US-China Medical Science, ISSN 1548-6648, USA,

Ghulam Naroo, Zulfiqar Ali, M. H. Shaji, Behrooz H. Vazirian, M. B. Falahkhir and M. Fikree

Abstract

Introduction:
Professional marathoners demonstrate abnormal rises in cardiac biomarkers and a spectrum of alterations in a 12-lead electrocardiogram (ECG). Such alterations are likely the consequence of athletic conditioning and represent another potential component of the athletic heart syndrome. It remains unclear, however, whether the exercise induced change in ECG or the increase in cardiac biomarkers in obviously healthy athletes is of any consequence. Abnormal levels of cardiac biomarkers in marathon runners may inevitably lead to a misdiagnosis.

Methods:
One hundred healthy marathon runners were enrolled in this study during Dubai Marathon, Jan 2010. ECGs were conducted and blood samples were collected 30 minutes before and less than 30 minutes after the race. A baseline renal function was obtained on these samples and a level of Troponin T (cTnT) was measured.

Results:
Thirteen percent (7/52) exhibited ECG abnormalities before and seventeen percent (9/52) after the race. There were no abnormal Troponin levels before the race but levels increased by an average of 14.28% after the race. This was not related to changes on the ECG. Only one participant with an abnormal Troponin level also had an abnormal pattern on ECG.

Conclusion:
Diagnostic biochemical tests are prone to changes following exercise. An increase in the cardiac biomarker Troponin T may be transient following marathon run. No correlation between the ECG pattern and a raised Troponin T has been found.

Introduction
It is a well documented fact that physical activity provides many benefits to cardiovascular health such as lowering blood pressure, improving lipid profile, modulating insulin resistance and decreasing overall mortality.[1] However, the occurrence of cardiac death and other adverse events post marathon run has also been well documented in the medical literature.[2-5] The data on the impact of screening programs is fairly limited and no randomized trial has ever been published in that direction. This may possibly reflect an extremely low incidence of sudden cardiac death in athletes, still it cannot entirely be ruled out that the possibility of preventing and perhaps even identifying athletes at risk of such adverse outcomes may very well exist.

Recent studies[6-11] have demonstrated the risks of exercise-associated cardiac damage and/or dysfunction, as evidenced by a rise in cardiac biomarkers. Of particular interest is the transient rise in activities of creatine kinase MB[12] following marathon run. Despite the evidence, there continues to be considerable debate over the consequence of such elevations in cardio specific markers such as troponin.[13, 14] That exercise can induce increases in cardiac Troponin T (cTnT) or cardiac Troponin I (cTnI) in obviously healthy athletes has been demonstrated in several studies in the past and has been the subject of a recent meta analysis[9] which concluded that nearly half the endurance athletes that have been studied have demonstrated a rise in cTnT.

The athletic heart syndrome is a well described phenomenon in the medical literature.[15] It is known to occur in trained athletes and is characterized by an enlargement of the heart muscle due to significant amounts of exercise. Studies have documented a variety of electrocardiographic changes in trained athletes, some of which include increased precordial R-wave or S-wave voltages, T-wave inversion and deep Q wave changes. Although this does raise the possibility of a pathological heart condition, it has more often been attributed to the cardiac morphological remodeling induced by the athletic condition.[16-20] Furthermore, the heart of an athlete may also demonstrate sinus bradycardia, right atrial enlargement, conduction delays like 1st and possibly 2nd degree heart block as well as early repolarization.[21, 22]

Although the need to further study such claims is recognized, the authors of this paper aim at studying the hypothesis that a rise in cTnT is related to myocardial damage in otherwise healthy athletes. We have, therefore, attempted to identify the relationship between cTnT and ECG in a group of athletes subjected to the vigorous exertion of a marathon.

Methods

One hundred participants were randomly enrolled in this study. Of the 400 marathon runners registered to run the 42 kilometer race at the annual Dubai Marathon, we chose the first 100 even numbers. The cosmopolitan nature of the city allowed us to recruit runners of 22 nationalities (including most of Western Europe, northern and central Africa and the Middle East). All runners provided written consent and completed a comprehensive screening form prior to the race. This was in the form of a questionnaire that included questions about current and past medical conditions, family history and the use of prescription medications, if any.

Blood samples were collected 30 minutes before and less than 30 minutes after the race. Samples were then sent to the Rashid Hospital Trauma Center laboratory and measured using electrochemiluminescence. Urea and Creatinine were also measured on all samples for the purpose of obtaining a baseline renal function. ECGs were also performed on all participants before and less than 30 minutes after the race.

Of the 100 enrolled participants, only 52 completed the study and underwent a post race electrocardiography. Of these 52, only 21 participants gave blood samples for a post race Troponin T level. Only men between the ages of 25 and 45 were included in this study. We felt including age among the variables was warranted since according to the American Heart Association guidelines abnormal ECG patterns in athletes below the age of 35 may be indicative of a congenital heart disease.[23] Of the 52 participants that did complete the study with follow up electrocardiograms, 20 were under the age of 35 and 32 were above the age of 35. Individuals with history of diabetes, hypertension or coronary artery disease were excluded. Also individuals with a positive family history of sudden death were not enrolled. The runners were divided into two groups. Regular runners (n=46) were defined as those with 12 weeks of preparation, 5 times a week with the longest run lasting 2 hours and aiming to run 20-40 miles per week. Beginners (n=6) were those under the 'get you round' program who had had no formal training.

ECGs performed on all participants were independently interpreted by three trained internal physicians and one trained emergency physician.

Results
Thirteen percent (7/52) exhibited ECG abnormalities before the race (Fig. 2). These included T wave inversions, incomplete Right Bundle Branch Block, early repolarization and LVH pattern. Post race this number rose to seventeen percent (9/52) (Fig. 3). Supraventricular tachycardias (SVT) were seen on both of these abnormal ECGs, although both were transient and neither required medical treatment. The pre-race ECGs of both these candidates showed normal sinus rhythm, no conduction defect or ST segment abnormality. Moreover both these participants were regular runners.

The cutoff value for Troponin T at our institution is ≤ 0.02 ng/mL. There was no raised Troponin identified on any of the samples sent before the race. After the race, however, Troponin levels increased by an average of 14.28% (Fig. 4a) but this was not associated with any ECG changes. These levels fell back to normal 8 hours post exercise.

The relationship between the raised Troponin and ECG patterns is illustrated in Fig. 5. Troponin T (TnT) was found positive in two runners with a normal ECG and one runner with an abnormal ECG (Fig 4b & 4c).

Discussion
Endurance exercise can induce increases in cardiac Troponin in healthy endurance athletes under special conditions (especially during endurance competitions), which do not represent irreversible myocardial damage but probably reversible transitory membrane leakage of cardiomyocytes and, therefore, seem to be without pathological significance. The exercise-induced releases of free cytoplasmic cardiac Troponins as well as B-type natriuretic peptide may induce cardiomyocytes' adaptation on endurance

exercise and modulate myocardial hypertrophy in otherwise healthy athletes. The underlying cellular mechanisms of exercise induced releases in cardiac Troponins and (N-terminal prohormone brain natriuretic peptide) B-type natriuretic peptide, however, have to be studied in the future to better understand their role in endurance exercise on the athletic heart.[13, 24, and 25]

The mechanisms responsible for post-exercise cTnT release are not known. Some have suggested that exercise-induced cardiac Troponin release precedes physiologic cardiac hypertrophy.[6, 8, 26, 27] Release of acidic and basic fibroblast growth factor (>FGF and AFGF, respectively) from the cytosol of cardiac myocytes has been demonstrated, occurring in response to membrane damage caused by an increase in the rate and force of cardiac contraction. Membrane damage, subsequent to an increased rate and force of cardiac contraction during endurance exercise, may prove a mechanism by which cytosolic Troponin is released into the circulation. High-intensity exercise, defined as high intensity running for 30 minutes, is also known to result in cTnI release.[28]

Although moderate aerobic exercise has documented health benefits,[1] the long term cardiac implications of repeated release of cTnT after multiple endurance events are less clear. Whether post-exercise cTnT release is related to micro-injury of the myocardium is presently not clear. Cross-sectional and longitudinal studies are required to further examine the causes and consequences of post-exercise cTnT release.

The limitations of this study include a small sample size. Also, Troponin levels at 24 hours were not performed but that is only because all abnormal Troponin levels had returned to normal within 8 hours. A creatinine clearance was substituted with a one time reading of Urea and Creatinine; therefore, it lacked a proper assessment of renal function. Finishing time of participants were not recorded. There is no financial support or conflict of interest.

Conclusion

In conclusion, many of the diagnostic biochemical tests on which we rely are affected by exercise. Physicians needs to be aware of these effects when interpreting results in clinical setting, so a full history is essential before interpreting any abnormality in these indices in order to avoid over-diagnosing marathon runners in particular with any pathology.

In contrast to acute myocardial infarction, increase in cTnT is only mild and of shorter duration in healthy athletes. Exercise-associated elevations in cTnT decreased well before the 8 hour mark so it may safely be concluded that values reach normal limits within such a time frame.

Our study shows no correlation between the ECG pattern and a raised Troponin. Blood tests in marathon runners may produce a raised Troponin post exercise. Screening of the athletic population of cardiovascular risk by doing 12 lead ECGs is not a proven diagnostic tool.

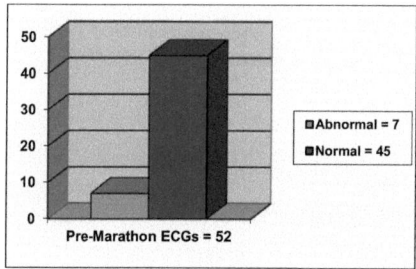

Figure 2: This graph shows the number of participants with abnormal ECGs prior to the race. These were mostly characterized by T wave inversion and LVH patterns.

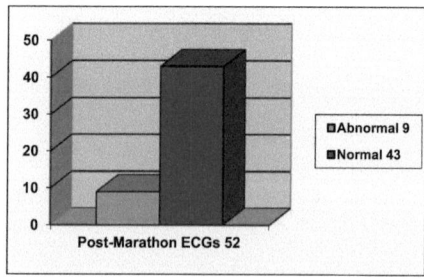

Beyond Pheidippides

Figure 3: This graph shows the number of participants with abnormal ECGs less than 30 minutes after the race.

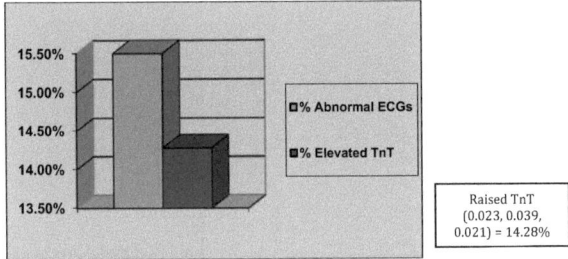

Figure 4a: This graph shows the number of participants with a raised TnT less than 30 minutes after the race.

Abnormal ECGs (9/52) = 17.3 %

Elevated TnT (3/21) = 14.3%

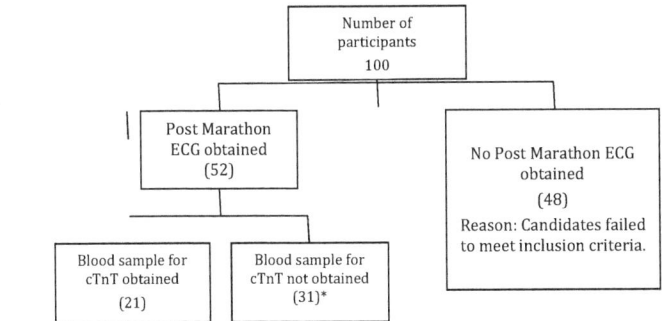

Figure 4b: Flowchart illustrating the number of participants ECGs and blood samples

were obtained on

* Candidates did not give follow up blood samples

Case no.	Age	Level of Training	Relevant History	Pre-race ECG	Post-race ECG	Pre-race TnT	Post-race TnT
152	41	Regular	None	Normal	Normal	Negative	0.023
44	39	Regular	None	Normal	Normal	Negative	0.039
118	38	Regular	None	LVH	LVH	Negative	0.021

Figure 4c: This table gives details of participants with an abnormally high TnT

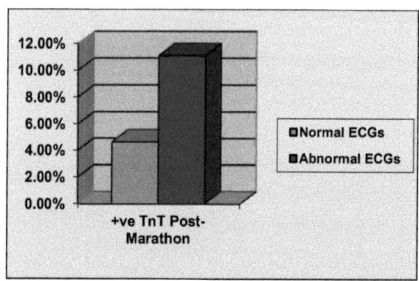

Figure 5: This graph illustrates the relationship between positive Troponin T values and post-marathon ECGs. TnT was found positive in two runners with normal ECG patterns and one with an abnormal ECG pattern.
Normal ECGs with Elevated Troponin = 4.65% (2/43)
Abnormal ECGs with Elevated Troponin = 11.1% (1/9)

Beyond Pheidippides

References

(1) Paffenbarger RS, Hyde RT, Wing AL, Lee I, Jung DL, Kampert JB. The Association of Changes in Physical-Activity Level and Other Lifestyle Characteristics with Mortality among Men. N.Engl.J.Med. 1993 02/25;328(8):538-545.

(2) Mittleman MA, Maclure M, Tofler GH, Sherwood JB, Goldberg RJ, Muller JE. Triggering of Acute Myocardial Infarction by Heavy Physical Exertion -- Protection against Triggering by Regular Exertion. N.Engl.J.Med. 1993 12/02;329(23):1677-1683.

(3) Maron BJ, Poliac LC, Roberts WO. Risk for sudden cardiac death associated with marathon running. J.Am.Coll.Cardiol. 1996 8;28(2):428-431.

(4) Ratliff NB, Harris KM, Smith SA, Tankh-Johnson M, Gornick CC, Maron BJ. Cardiac arrest in a young marathon runner. Lancet 2002 Aug 17;360(9332):542.

(5) Thompson PD. The cardiovascular complications of vigorous physical activity. Arch.Intern.Med. 1996 Nov 11;156(20):2297-2302.

(6) Koller A. Exercise-induced increases in cardiac troponins and prothrombotic markers. Med.Sci.Sports Exerc. 2003 Mar;35(3):444-448.

(7) Scharhag J, Shave R, George K, Whyte G, Kindermann W. "Exercise-induced increases in cardiac troponins in endurance athletes: a matter of exercise duration and intensity?". Clin.Res.Cardiol. 2008 Jan;97(1):62-3; author reply 61.

(8) Scharhag J, Urhausen A, Schneider G, Herrmann M, Schumacher K, Haschke M, et al. Reproducibility and clinical significance of exercise-induced increases in cardiac troponins and N-terminal pro brain natriuretic peptide in endurance athletes. Eur.J.Cardiovasc.Prev.Rehabil. 2006 Jun;13(3):388-397.

(9) Shave R, George KP, Atkinson G, Hart E, Middleton N, Whyte G, et al. Exercise-induced cardiac troponin T release: a meta-analysis. Med.Sci.Sports Exerc. 2007 Dec;39(12):2099-2106.

(10) Shave R, George K, Gaze D. The influence of exercise upon cardiac biomarkers: a practical guide for clinicians and scientists. Curr.Med.Chem. 2007;14(13):1427-1436.

(11) Whyte G, Stephens N, Senior R, George K, Shave R, Wilson M, et al. Treat the patient not the blood test: the implications of an increase in cardiac troponin after prolonged endurance exercise. British Journal of Sports Medicine September 01;41:613-615.

(12) Ohman EM, Teo KK, Johnson AH, Collins PB, Dowsett DG, Ennis JT, et al. Abnormal cardiac enzyme responses after strenuous exercise: alternative diagnostic aids. Br.Med.J.(Clin.Res.Ed) 1982 Nov 27;285(6354):1523-1526.

(13) Siegel AJ, Lewandrowski EL, Chun KY, Sholar MB, Fischman AJ, Lewandrowski KB. Changes in cardiac markers including B-natriuretic peptide in runners after the Boston marathon. Am.J.Cardiol. 2001 Oct 15;88(8):920-923.

(14) Siegel AJ, Sholar M, Yang J, Dhanak E, Lewandrowski KB. Elevated serum cardiac markers in asymptomatic marathon runners after competition: is the myocardium stunned? Cardiology 1997 Nov-Dec;88(6):487-491.

(15) John T. Lohr. Athletic heart syndrome. In: Jacqueline L. Longe, editor. 3ed ed. 2006.

(16) Venerando A, Rulli V. Frequency Morphology and Meaning of the Electrocardiographic Anomalies found in Olympic Marathon Runners and Walkers. J.Sports Med.Phys.Fitness 1964 Sep;50:135-141.

(17) Hanne-Paparo N, Wendkos MH, Brunner D. T wave abnormalities in the electrocardiograms of top-ranking athletes without demonstrable organic heart disease. Am.Heart J. 1971 Jun;81(6):743-747.

(18) Lichtman J, O'Rourke RA, Klein A, Karliner JS. Electrocardiogram of the athlete. Alterations simulating those of organic heart disease. Arch.Intern.Med. 1973 Nov;132(5):763-770.

(19) Maron BJ, Pelliccia A. The heart of trained athletes: cardiac remodeling and the risks of sports, including sudden death. Circulation 2006 Oct 10;114(15):1633-1644.

(20) Huston TP, Puffer JC, Rodney WM. The athletic heart syndrome. N.Engl.J.Med. 1985 Jul 4;313(1):24-32.

(21) Thompson PD. Cardiovascular adaptations to marathon running: the marathoner's heart. Sports Med. 2007;37(4-5):444-447.

(22) Tunstall Pedoe DS. Marathon cardiac deaths: the london experience. Sports Med. 2007;37(4-5):448-450.

(23) Maron BJ, Thompson PD, Puffer JC, McGrew CA, Strong WB, Douglas PS, et al. Cardiovascular preparticipation screening of competitive athletes: addendum: an addendum to a statement for health professionals from the Sudden Death Committee (Council on Clinical Cardiology) and the Congenital Cardiac Defects Committee (Council on Cardiovascular Disease in the Young), American Heart Association. Circulation 1998 Jun 9;97(22):2294.

(24) Kratz A, Lewandrowski KB, Siegel AJ, Chun KY, Flood JG, Van Cott EM, et al. Effect of marathon running on hematologic and biochemical laboratory parameters, including cardiac markers. Am.J.Clin.Pathol. 2002 Dec;118(6):856-863.

(25) Siegel AJ, Stec JJ, Lipinska I, Van Cott EM, Lewandrowski KB, Ridker PM, et al. Effect of marathon running on inflammatory and hemostatic markers. Am.J.Cardiol. 2001 Oct 15;88(8):918-20, A9.

(26) Koller A. Postexercise increases in cardiac troponin T and brain natriuretic peptide. Med.Sci.Sports Exerc. 2004 Apr;36(4):736; author response 737.

(27) Shave R, Dawson E, Whyte G, George K, Nimmo M, Layden J, et al. The impact of prolonged exercise in a cold environment upon cardiac function. Med.Sci.Sports Exerc. 2004 Sep;36(9):1522-1527.

(28) Shave R, Ross P, Low D, George K, Gaze D. Cardiac troponin I is released following high-intensity short-duration exercise in healthy humans. Int.J.Cardiol. 2010 Jan 13

2.2. MARATHON RUNNING AS A CAUSE OF TROPONIN ELEVATION; A SYSTEMIC REVIEW AND META-ANALYSIS.

Journal of International Cardiology
Volume 23, Issue 5, 443-450, Oct 2010.
Steven Regwan D.O, Edward a. Hulten MD, Jenifer Slim D.O. MD, Todd C.Villines MD, Ahmad M. Slim MD.

A total of 939 participants met the criteria for inclusion in this analysis. Medline database was searched through ovoid search service in humans older than 18 years of age and published from 1983- Dec 2008.

Results: 16 studies reported cardiac Troponin changes prior to and immediately following the race[1-15]. In these series 6/940 (0.6%) had non negative Troponin before the marathon compared to 579/936 (62%) with positive Troponin after the race.

Despite some limitations of the study it provided insight into the average reported incidence of elevated Troponin levels after the marathon race.

Conclusion: Given the current data available, there is statistically significant incidence of exercise induced asymptomatic Troponin release among the marathon runners. This is consistent with cytosolic release theory and not myocardial injury. It is based on short time to peak and resolution within 24 hours.

References:

1. Cummins P, Young A, Auckland ML, et al. Comaprison of serum cardiac kinase, creatine kinase-MB isoenzyme, tropomysin, myoglobin and C-reactive protein release in marathon runners: Cardiac or skeletal muscle trauma. Eur J Clin Invest 1987;17:317-324

2. Koller A, Mair J, Mayr M et al. Diagnosis of myocardial injury in marathon runners. Ann N Y Ascad Sci 1995;752:234-235.

3. Lucia A, Moran P, Perez M, et al. Short term effects of marathon running in master runners: No evidence of myocardial injury. Int J Sports Med 1999;20:482-486.

4. Lucia A, Serratosa L, Saborido A, et al. Short term effects of marathon running: No evidence of cardiac dysfunction. Med Sci sports Exerc 1999;31:1414-1421.

5. Kratz A, Lewandrowski KB, Siegel AJ, et al. Effects of marathon running on hematologic and biochemical laboratory parameters, including cardiac markers. Am J Clin Pathol 2002;118:856-863.

6. Herrmann M, Scharhag J, Miclea M, et al. Post race kinetics of cardiac troponin T and I and N-terminal pro-brain natriuretic peptide in marathon runners. Clin Chem 2003;49:831-834.

7. Fortescue EB, Shin Ay, Greens Ds, et al. Cardiac troponin increases among runners in the Boston marathon. Ann Emerg Med 2007;49:137-143.

8. Dawson Ea, Whyte GP, Black MA, et al. Changes in vascular and cardiac function after prolonged strenuous exercise in humans. J Appl Physiol 2008;105:1562-1568.

9. Siegel AJ, Lewandrowski KB, Strauss HW, et al. Normal post-race antimyosin myocardial scintigraph in asymptomatic marathon runners with elevated serum creatine kinase MB isoenzyme and troponin T levels. Cardiology 1995;86:451-456.

10. Apple FS,Quist HE, Otto AP, et al. Release characteristics of cardiac biomarkers and ischemia –modified albumin as measured by the albumin cobalt-binding test after a marathon race. Clin Chem 2002;48:1097-1100.

11. Whyte GP, George K, Shave RE, et al. Impact of marathon running on cardiac structure and function in recreational runners. Clin Sci 2005;108:73-80.

12. Shave Re, Whyte GP, George K, et al. Prolonged exercise should be considered alongside typical symptoms of acute myocardial infarction when evaluating increase in cardiac troponin T. Heart 2005;91:1219-1220.

13. Middelton N, Shave RE, Keith G, et al. Novel application of flow propagation velocity and ischemia-modified albumin in analysis of post exercise cardiac function in man. Exp physiol 2006;91:511-519.

14. Saenz Aj, Lee-Lewandrowski E, Wood MJ, et al.. Measurement of a plasma stroke biomarker panel and cardiac troponin T in marathon runners before and after the 2005 Boston marathon. Am J Clin Pathol 2006;126:185-189.

2.3. INFLUENCE OF HALF MARATHON RACE UPON CARDIAC TROPONIN T RELEASE IN ADOLESCENT RUNNERS.

Current Medicinal chemistry, 2011;18: 3452-3456.
J. Nie, K.P George, T.K. Tong, D. Gaze, Y. Tian, H. Lin, and Q. Shi.

A total of 63 adolescent runners were included in this study. A cardiological examination of all participants was carried out aweek prior to the race. They all completed the 21-Km race at the maximum pace. Blood samples were taken pre- race, immediate post race, four hours post race and 24 hours post race.

Results: It demonstrated that post exercise cardiac troponin T was almost universal among the runners. The relevant percentage of samples above clinical cut off were high (90% and 70% of the adolescents had cTnT concentration above 0.01ug/L detection level and 0.05 ug/L clinical threshold respectively) and individual data reached 1.36 ug/L. It was also found that the individuals with less than three years of training had increased incidence of changes in cTnT levels.

In this study the key finding was high number of detectable cTnT values all these runners. Recent data [1] suggested that exercise duration and intensity are essential factors in eliciting the release of cTnT and cTnI after a prolonged exertion[2]. In current study 51/63(81%) adolescent athletes had cTnT values above 0.03 ug/L post exercise.

The mechanism which lead to cTnT release is not well known. It was previously speculated that cTnT release during endurance sports is mediated through myocardial stunning[3], the ischemic development of blebs[4] and transient changes in membrane permeability[5].

It is important to point some technical limitations in the current study i.e. firstly it consisted of competitive adolescent runners the maturational age across the group will likely have varied considerably but there was no direct measure of this. Secondly most of our athletes were male and as such sex comparison is limited by unbalanced numbers. Further studies should assess these issues.

Beyond Pheidippides

Conclusion: In this study of a relatively large group of runners completed 21-km run, it was found that 90% of those had some degree of cTnT level increase, whereas 70% of them showed elevated cTnT level above 0.05ugm/L. In addition adolescents with less training experience were more prone to greater release of cTnT.

References:

1. Fu F, Nie J, Tong TK. Serum cardiac troponin T in adolescent runners: Effects of exercise intensity and duration. Int. J. Sports Med 2009;30(3):168-172.

2. Serrano-Ostariz E, Terreros-Blanco JL, Legaz-Arrese A, George K,Shave R, et al. The impact of exercise duration and intensity on release of cardiac biomarkers. Scand. J. Med. Sci. Sports 2009;21(2):244-249.

3. Starnes JW, Bowles DK. Role of exercise in the cause and prevention of cardiac dysfunction. Exerc. Sport Sci. Rev. 1995;23:349-373.

4. Hickman PE, Potter JM, Aroney C, Koerbin G. et al. Cardiac troponin may be released by ischemia alone, without necrosis. Clin. Chim. Acta 2010;411(5-6):318-323.

5. Neumayr G, Pfister R, Mitterbauer G, Maurer A, Gaenzer H, et al. Effect of the "Race across Alps" in elite cyclists on plasma cardiac troponins I and T. Am. J. Cardiol. 2002;89(4):484-486.

2.4. CARDIAC TROPONIN IN YOUNG MARATHON RUNNERS:

American Journal of Cardiology 2012 ,Volume 110, Issue 4:594-598.
Natthapon Traiperm Msc, Hannes Gatterer Msc, Maria Wille Msc and Burtscher

Forty young runners (20 healthy male and 20 female) participated in this study. They were between 13-17 years of age. Blood sample were collected before, immediately after and 24 hours post race to determine and compare the cTnT levels. Thirty seven runners completed the race without any adverse medical event. All runners were advised to run at individual pace conforming to their running ability. They were continuously supervised by a medical doctor. EKG was done before the start of the race and it didn't show any abnormality.

Results:
Thirty seven runners completed the race whereas three of them were dropped out due to shoes problems. Mean values for cardiac troponin did not differ between boys and girls. There were statistically significant changes over time. In 30 (81%) runners the cTnT level exceeded the upper reference limit of 0.01ng/ml in immediate post race sample. One had values higher than the Acute Myocardial Infarction (AMI) cutoff for cTnT (0.1ng/ml) and 2 subjects had higher values AMI cutoff for cTnI (0.5ng/ml). Twenty four hours post race troponin levels reverted to normal in all participants.

The main findings in this study was the immediate post race cardiac troponin levels exceeded the upper reference limit of 0.01ng/ml for cTnT being indicative of possible myocardial injury[1][2]. Cardiac Troponin levels have been frequently investigated after endurance sports like marathons,[3][4][5] ultramarathons,[6][7] triathalons,[8][9] and cycling races[10]. Most studies have shown an increased levels of cardiac troponin in immediate post race period. Fu et al[11] found increased levels of cTnT and cTnI immediately. 45 minutes and 90 minutes after treadmill running. Tian et al[12] also found increased values after 21 km run. Although the cardiac troponin levels have been related to the intensity and duration of the exercise in adolescents [11][12], results of this study indicate that running an entire marathon leads to same response as in half marathon run.

Cardiac magnetic resonance imaging in recent studies have suggested that increase in cardiac troponins are not caused by myocardial injury [13]. Therefore it seems likely that increased cardiac troponins after strenuous exercise is a physiological rather than a pathological response[14].

Conclusion:
This was the first study which included equal number of male and female participants. Average increase of cTnT and cTnI level did not differ in between the sexes. More than 80% of the participants demonstrated the increase in the level of cardiac troponin immediate post race which returned to base line within 24 hours. None of the runners exhibited the adverse medical effects during or after the race.

References:

1. Apple FS, Quist HE, Doyle PJ and Murakami MM. Plasma 99th percentile reference limits for cardiac troponin and creatine kinase MB mass for use with European society of Cardiology/American college of Cardiology consensus recommendations. Clin C 2003;49:1331-1336.

2. Scharhag J, George K, Shave R, et al. Exercise associated increase in cardiac biomarkers. Med Sci Sports Exerc. 2008;10:1408-1415.

3. Fortescue EB, Shin AY, Greenes DS, et al. Cardiac troponin increase among runners in Boston marathon. Ann Emerg Med 2007;49:137-143.

4. Koller A, Sumann G, Griesmacher A, et al. Cardiac troponins after a downhill marathon. Int J Cardiol 2008;129"449-452.

5. Hubble KM, Fatovich DB, Grasko JM and Vasikaran SD. Cardiac troponin increase in marathons stud. Med J Aust 2009;190:91-93.

6. Ohba H, Takada H, Musha H, et al. Effects of prolonged strenuous exercise on plasma level of atrial natriuretic peptide and brain natriuretic peptide in healthy men. Am Heart J 2001;141:751-758.

7. Musha H, Nagashima J, Awaya T, et al. Myocardial injury in a 100-km ultramarathon. Curr Ther Res 1997;58:587-593.

8. Cleave P, Boswell TD, Speedy DB, and Boswell DR. Plasma Cardiac troponin concentrations after extreme exercise. Clin Chem 2001;47:608-610.

9. Rifai N, Douglas PS, O'Toole M, et al. Cardiac troponin T and I, echocardiographic (correction of echocardiographic) wall motion analysis, and ejection fractions in athletes participating in Hawaii Ironman Trathlon. Am J Cardiol 1999;83:1085-1089.

10. Neumayr G, Pfister R, Mitterbauer G, et al. Effect of the "Race across the Alps" in elite cyclists on plasma cardiac troponins I and T. Am J Cardiol 2002;89:484-486.

11. Fu F, Nie J and Tong Tk. Serum cardiac troponin T in adolescent runners: effects of exercise intensity and duration. Int J Sports Med 2009;30:168-172.

12. Tian Y, Nie J, Tong TK, Gao Q, et al. Changes in serum cardiac troponins following a 21-km run in junior male runners. J Sports Med Phys Fitnessfit 2009;46:481-486.

13. Trivax Je, Franklin BA, Goldstein JA, et al. Acute cardiac effects of marathon running. J Appl Physiol 2010;108:1148-1153.

14. Nie J, Tong TK, George K, et al. Resting and post exercise serum biomarkers of cardiac and skeletal muscle damage in adolescent runners. Scand J Med Sci Sports 2011;21:625-629.

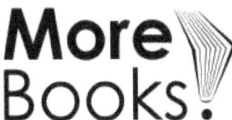
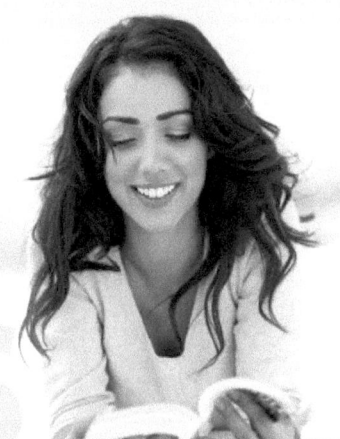

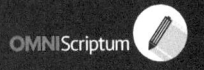

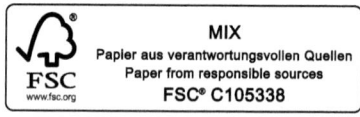

Printed by Books on Demand GmbH, Norderstedt / Germany